Triple F
Fifty Fit and Fabulous
Proof that Fitness is for Any Age

Sharon Simmons

Triple F: Fifty, Fit, and Fabulous
Proof That Fitness Is for Any Age

FIRST EDITION 2009
Printed in USA

ISBN: 1-4392-4311-5
ISBN-13: 9781439243114
Library of Congress Control Number: 2009905272

Visit www.booksurge.com to order additional copies.

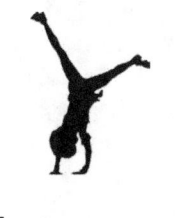

Foreward

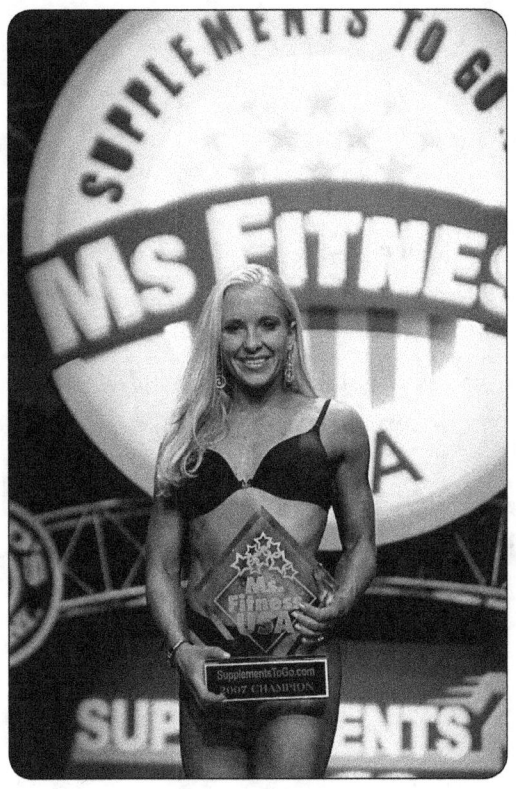

As former Ms. Fitness USA, I understand how much time, energy and commitment goes into leading a healthy lifestyle. I met Sharon Simmons when she began competing at the age of 50--she is proof that Fitness is for Any Age. She is truly TRIPLE "F" - Fifty, Fit, and Fabulous!

Cara Kokenes Samson
Ms. Fitness USA 2007
Executive Director for Miss Chicago

In Loving Memory

The right way is the hard way, and the wrong way is easy.
—Larry Simmons, father-in-law

Petey: My friend, companion, and loving blind
Miniature Schnauzer for eleven wonderful years.

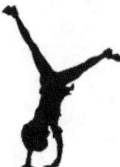

Table of Contents

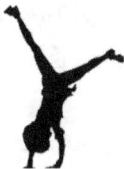

Purpose of Triple F—
What to Expect

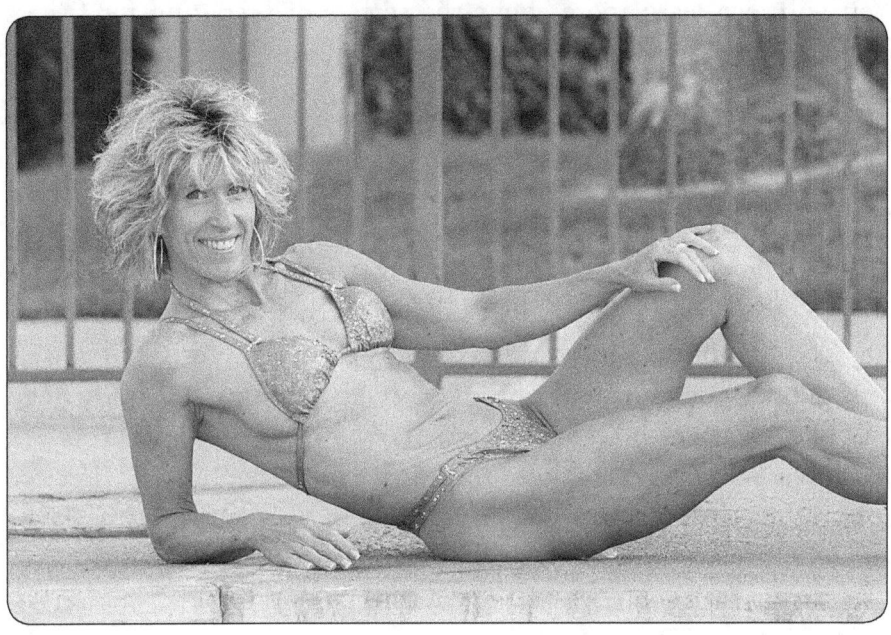

Do you want to feel better, look better, and live longer? Then keep reading! For all of my life, I have been striving to live a healthier lifestyle, which has provided me with the wonderful opportunity to look better and be *fit at any age*—and hopefully live a longer life, too. In the following chapters, you will be able to develop a basic plan for a healthier lifestyle and come to believe that you CAN DO THIS, too. Make a commitment to a better you, and I will commit to help you.

During the course of reading and digesting this book, you are going to find out some of my secrets for not only looking younger but feeling younger too. What you will not find is a quick, easy fix for challenges; but what you will discover is a viable course to leading a healthy lifestyle *not* surrounded by diets and drugs. You will learn about the author, nutrition, exercise, supplements, and goal setting along with the challenges.

Think about how nervous you are when you make a decision to begin an exercise program and walk into the gym that first day. You feel like everyone is looking at just you. You feel like you need to lose weight and be in shape just to join a gym! It is a very intimidating feeling. I will teach you how to overcome those dreaded gym fears. You will also learn more about the secrets of preparing for fitness competitions and some of the down and dirty useful *tricks* of a fitness competitor. Then you will be able to read actual testimonials of everyday people in their pursuit of being fit at any age.

Qualifications

Why am I qualified to tell you how to lead a healthier lifestyle and be fit at any age? Well, let's talk about that. I have been exercising now for almost fifty years— literally. I have been studying exercise and nutrition for most of those years, because feeling really good and looking good interest me. Don't they interest you, too? You will learn more about my background in the next chapter, but here are some of my qualifications so you will feel more comfortable with the things that we will share throughout the book. If you have questions, you can always contact me at www.FitnessAnyAge.com.

- Certified Personal Trainer
- Certified Nutritional Specialist
- Featured in *Ms. Fitness Magazine*, "Fit Over Forty," Summer 2009
- Appearances in *Ms. Fitness Magazine, 2006, 2007, 2008, 2009,* and advertising the *Ms. Fitness USA* Fitness Show (www.msfitness.com)
- Featured in full-page article, *Citizen's Gazette,* "Training for Fitness Competitions over 50!" August 2007
- Featured in infomercial, "Hot on Health and Beauty," 2008, Dallas, Texas

- Guest speaker on *Channel 5 Health Fit Expo*, Dallas Convention Center, "What Does Fitness Mean to Me?" February 2007
- Spokesperson at numerous fitness events across the United States
- Master of Arts in Organizational Management
- Bachelor's Degree in Business Management
- Associate's Degree of Applied Science in Mid-Management

Pride, Passion, and Commitment

With your pride, passion, and commitment, I am confident that I can accompany you on this journey to a healthier lifestyle and coach you on ways to feel younger and look younger. I am passionate about the subject of *fitness*, and I firmly believe that fitness is for any age. Remember, you have to first believe in yourself and who you are and have faith you can accomplish your goals. Just know you have someone who understands and will support you—me.

OK. Let's get started! Turn the page to learn more about me and some of my secrets to fitness at whatever age you are. Make this your *defining moment*, and then make a commitment towards health and fitness.

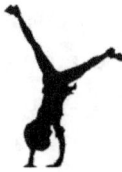

Getting to Know Sharon

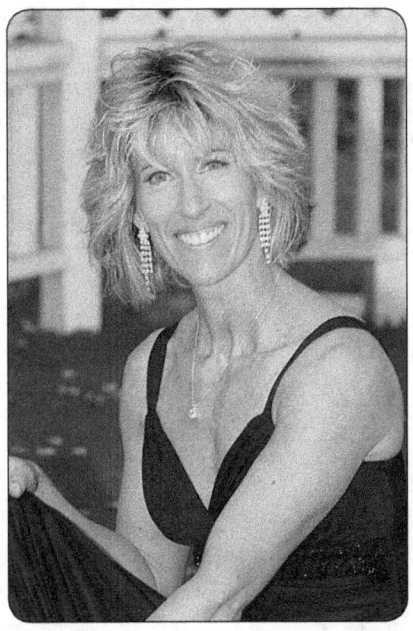

Who is Sharon Simmons anyway? Before you and I begin to share our lives, I think it is very important to get to know each other. I'll start off by telling you a little about how I grew up. Let's go back over fifty years to Nashville, Tennessee, where a little girl was the firstborn of three children and a single mom who worked as a waitress to feed her family. My mother was the oldest of nine children, had barely a ninth grade education, and was married at just fifteen years of age. My father passed away after many abusive years of alcoholism. Through it all, I never lost my dreams of attending college, making lots of money, and raising a family of my own—the American dream, right?

Well, things didn't quite turn out that way for me. In fact, I did things a little backwards. My family was poor growing up; my two brothers and I had lots of gravy and biscuits, no meat, and sugary cereals as our main diet because of a very low family income. Our father would pull a three-day drunk and then come home and pawn whatever piece of furniture or household equipment he could to purchase alcohol. The memory still lingers of him asleep at the small kitchen table with his head lying in his plate of food! That's right—that's what I said—in his food. The three of us, and Mom, were all too afraid to say anything to wake him because he was so violent and mean that he would hit us or break the furniture. He would even make us wash his feet in a bowl of water after not showering for three days; to this day, I can't stand the smell of *Limburger cheese.*

My father was so mean to every living creature that I used to catch the cockroaches and push them through the cracks in the house just so he wouldn't kill them, too. I remember eating things he killed: all kinds of fish, squirrel, groundhogs, turtles, and one time, even a small goat. He brought it home alive, and another man hit the goat in the face. This memory haunts me to this day, and I cannot erase the sorrow and terror I felt for this precious little animal.

The fire department just around the corner provided my brothers and me with gently used holiday gifts and food for our holiday dinner. To this day, I have a large, tattered Cinderella book in my cedar chest given to me by one of the firemen *in the same condition* that he presented it to me over forty years ago. One happy year, all three of us received a brand new bike for Christmas, and we rode all over the neighborhood every day and what seemed to be all night, too. Mr. and Mrs. Green, my mother's customers at Varello's Restaurant, gave mom one hundred dollars to spend for Christmas. They took a liking to her and felt sorry for her situation and wanted to help.

In one house where we lived in the *attic*, which had been converted into a small apartment, I recall watching large rats run up the walls and across the ceilings. I bet you didn't know rats could do that. It wasn't really that scary or odd to us at the time, because we had actually become used to this type of living condition. One time, an injured rat ran across my brother's foot and left blood on it. Mom got very scared when she thought the rat had bitten my brother. The apartment had slanted ceilings, and we would sneak into a side room and peer down between the support beams to the apartment below to watch the man downstairs walk around in his underwear—remember "tightie-whities"? Yuck.

There was another apartment where we lived for a few months that was right next door to Miss Nancy of *Romper Room*—how cool was that! I don't know if any of you remember *Romper Room* or not, but it was like meeting a movie star. The cool thing about living there was that it wasn't too far from Grandma (on my Dad's side) and we could walk over on Wednesday night just to watch *Lost in Space*. "Danger, Will Robinson."

Then the obvious thing happened; we were evicted for non-payment of rent, and all of our worldly belongings were on the street when I got home from school. So we moved just down the street from our school, Lockeland Elementary. I was known as the Queen of Tetherball, and the kids called me Flea because I was so small and skinny. The principal of the school, Mr. Rutherford, would allow my brothers and me to "shop" for free in their room of donated clothing so we would have school clothes. I still remember my sixth grade teacher, Mr. Marable, reading about the Tar Baby and holding square dancing lessons in class. This was too fun and a great memory. Ironically, now the *old neighborhood* is Nashville's Historical District, paved with brick streets and considered beautiful.

My first year of junior high at East Junior High School on Gallatin Road was a tough year for me; we couldn't afford sports, clothes, or even food. Everything had to be donated to our family. Right after my thirteenth birthday, a friend of my mother paid for plane tickets to have the family flown to Texas to live with our Granny (on my mom's side) to escape our father's drinking and violent rages. I knew something was up when the lady told me I would be allowed to take my two guinea pigs with me on the plane for a ride. In spite of all of the years of abuse to our mother, my brothers, and me, and even though I was so totally afraid of my father, I cried with sadness at leaving him.

We waited to escape until he was admitted to the hospital for bleeding ulcers from alcohol. We had to leave in the middle of the day with only the *clothes on our backs* to escape, because he would have killed all of us—we knew it. After all, I had witnessed my father hold a shotgun to my mother's neck, threatening to kill her right in front of my brothers and me, so this escape was necessary. I know this sounds terrible to some, but our lives were surreal and a living hell.

My father passed away at forty-six years of age from cirrhosis of the liver a few years later. I recall speaking with him on the telephone; he begged me to come to see him. I told him, "I wouldn't walk across the street to your funeral." Looking back, I really do not recommend this; it was not the right thing to do no matter how much hurt was bottled up inside me.

I thought living with Granny and three other older teenagers, our aunts and uncles, was so awful. It was sad to leave my friends, clothes, school—everything we knew that was normal, even though it wasn't worth a dime. After a few months, we moved back to Tennessee and moved in with another family for protection from our father before he became very ill and passed away. This wasn't too bad, although we still didn't have any money, so I wasn't allowed to compete in any school sports. I was still very active after school practicing with some of the athletes and coaches on the balance beam and uneven parallel bars. They knew I didn't have any formal training, but they were nice enough to help. I also loved to dance, especially in front of a mirror. I excelled in the school-required sports such as track, dodge ball, tetherball, softball, etc. I even received the Presidential All-Around Sports Badge in school for excelling in all school-required sports. Boy, could I run and throw a baseball!

Then I became interested in boys—older boys. My mother wasn't around very much anyway; she once worked three jobs just to support the family. My brothers and I did basically what we wanted to do but didn't get into too much trouble. I never smoked or drank or did drugs—nothing like that. I still remember riding my bike with my two brothers down by the creek side catching crawdads. This is actually very funny, because while others may eat crawdads—that seems terrible to me, and heartless—I released them back into the creek.

I completed junior high, and after ninth grade, our family moved back to Texas. My mother married a man twelve years her junior, which made him only twenty-one years of age—I was fifteen! You can see the issue here. I gave this guy hell; he later became my hero.

I attended high school in Texas, and it was still very rocky for the family financially. The older kids would make fun of my clothes, and I didn't have a lot of friends but was very smart in school. In fact, I excelled with straight A's, plus I was very athletic. I played all of the school-sponsored sports such as volleyball and softball, and I was one of the fastest stars in the relay races. I would meet my friend on the weekends and play tennis with a borrowed racket.

In fact, I was playing tennis in the middle of the street when I told my brother that my stomach was upset and I had to go inside. Very quickly I discovered the upset stomach was no flu bug. I was pregnant at the young age of sixteen and had to get married to the baby's father, who was only seventeen. I only needed two credits remaining to graduate, so I went to summer school and completed my high school education, again with straight A's. No one knew I was pregnant other than my family.

The baby's father and I moved out on our own to raise our new daughter—babies raising babies. This lasted three short years. From there, it was a child mother struggling to make it on her own, going from one relationship to another. I never lost hope of the dreams of a higher education and a deep love of fitness. I would work out in my living room to music because I still didn't have any money to join a health club. Additionally, I entered the local junior college and began taking one class at a time to continue my education. I was always a tiny little thing with loads of energy—I had to be, in order to raise a daughter on my own.

Then I married again and had a son—a very rocky marriage that lasted only six years. Still struggling with this situation, I remained focused on education and working out. I continued working out so much that I got stronger and stronger. I also kept going to school.

I met a wonderful man and later got married, and then I completed my associate's degree in mid-management. With the support of my husband, I continued my education while working full time until completing my second degree, a bachelor's in business management. In spite of how difficult it was working and raising a family—not to mention my blind miniature schnauzer, Petey—I completed graduate school with a master's degree in organizational management at the age of fifty.

I achieved this while working full time managing commercial office buildings with a full staff and raising a son, ultimately putting him through college successfully for his criminal justice degree. My daughter went on to pursue her career and is now happily married and raising two incredible children. She serves on several educational boards and is heavily involved in her children's schools and sport activities while working full-time. High energy levels seem to run in my family.

I never lost sight of my love of fitness. At the age of fifty, I decided completing my degree wasn't enough of a challenge, so I competed in my first fitness competition. In fact, I competed in four competitions *during my first year*. It all began when I experienced a defining moment one day in kickboxing class when looking at pictures of the instructor from a competition. I decided at that moment that this would be my next challenge, and then I took steps to accomplish the new goal. A later chapter discusses defining moments and how important they are to goals.

Believe me; this was not easy at the age of fifty. Since I never took gymnastics, dance, cheerleading, or had any other formal training, it was extra challenging for a woman my age to not only learn choreography but the physical aspect of competing in fitness. Quite frankly, I was a bit stiff. I had to work extra hard stretching and pointing my toes when performing high kicks.

My husband recalls when I came home one day from work and proudly said, "Honey, I'm going to compete in a fitness competition." Knowing how goal-oriented his wife is, he simply said, "OK." After my first choreography session, I came home close to tears saying, "I can't perform the cheerleading moves." Then I approached my dance teacher, Micaela Brigida (founder and president of Orizon, an International Creative Movement) from my fitness club and asked her if she would come out of retirement to teach me a fitness routine.

Micaela's motto is that dancing isn't about being the best but on the contrary is the foundation of inspiring others to accomplish the impossible at times: joy, happiness, laughter, peace, love, higher purpose, courage, unity, compassion, friendship, family, sharing, giving, receiving, self-motivation, faith, peace, believing in oneself, and the understanding of oneness of our higher power. She agreed to help, saying it was because of my obvious dedication and love for fitness. This lady believed in me and was able to teach me the very first routine that I had ever performed—it was to "These Boots Are Made for Walking." It brought tears to my eyes when she said, "You have learned your first element." Then I said, "I have an element." I didn't even know what an element was! But that was only the beginning of my learning curve. The struggle of learning about proper nutrition for a fitness competitor—that's another whole ballgame. Whew!

My very first fitness competition was incredibly unreal: in Las Vegas, Nevada, at the Ms. Fitness USA Fitness Show, on a stage at the Rio Hotel. I performed the routine, spoke in an evening gown, and participated in the physique competition with the other competitors. It was like heaven!

My second competition was with the Fitness America Pageant in Ft. Worth, Texas, in the Open Fitness and Fitness Model categories. My daughter proudly nicknamed me Triple F: Fifty, Fit, and Fabulous. I took second place in both categories. Ladies and gentlemen, this is saying something. At the young age of fifty, I placed second in open categories with girls ranging from twenty to thirty-six years old. The announcer kept calling me Triple X instead of Triple F; I think he was drinking more than a soft drink in that large paper cup. Then he actually announced me as "Grandma" as I walked out on stage. To this day, I can still hear my husband yelling, and my son screaming, "MOM!" It was a feeling like no other—it was awesome! I was hooked.

People ask, "Why do you do this?" and I respond, "Because I can." My husband is completely supportive of my goals and ambitions and has even begun his own fitness program and looks fantastic. My son competed in his first National Physique Committee (NPC) competition and placed second in his weight category. My mom doesn't completely understand the whole fitness competition thing, but she watches all the videos and shows my pictures to everyone. My company has been very supportive and announced one of the big wins at their annual meeting. When I'm in the middle of a training season, the people in the gym don't quite understand the "weird" training moves that I do or the strange nutrition plan I eat on a daily basis, but they watch and ask questions.

This goal has not been easy for me, but it has been every bit rewarding. I am all about the statement "Fitness Is for Any Age." It is not restrictive based on how much money you have or how old you are. It is about a burning, sincere desire to achieve results and live a healthier life. I firmly believe you can accomplish anything in life that you want, as long as you want it badly enough and you believe! It is about having a firm belief in yourself and what you can do. It is a passion that comes from within and the pursuit of a healthy lifestyle. We each only have one body, and we need to take care of it. It's not about where you've been; it's about where you're going.

So please keep reading and learn. You can do this. Set your goal—whatever that might be—education, a new career, or achieving a healthier lifestyle. **Never allow anyone to set your limitations—**make a decision and the sky is the limit. *Just do it!* Fitness is for Any Age.

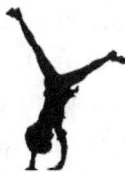

Exercise at Any Age

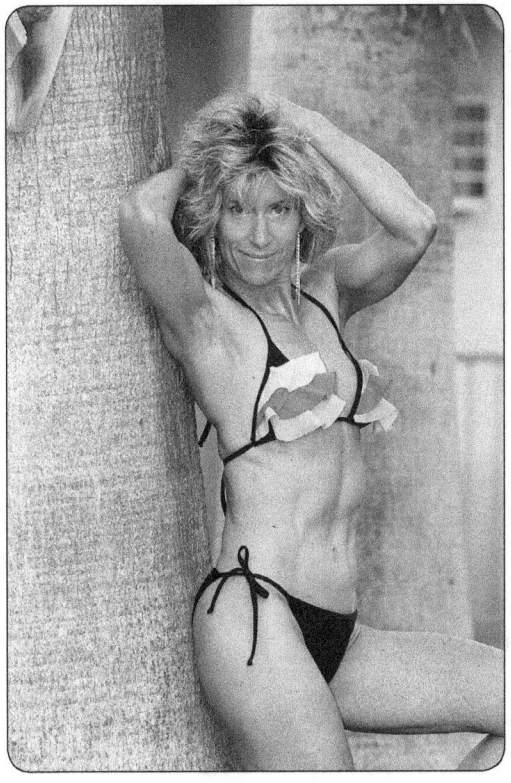

You will hear this same message throughout the book. There are basically two secrets to Fitness at Any Age: Good Nutrition (a variety of non-processed foods), and Exercise (get your body moving). That's it! The key to keeping your mind, body, and spirit healthy and fit is to EXERCISE.

Everyone wants to think it is as simple as buying one of those crazy machines you see on TV. This reminds me of that movie where the guy picks up the hitchhiker, and the guy is really nuts. He is telling the driver about a new invention he has, "The 7-Minute Abs." The driver asks him why it isn't called the "5-Minute Abs" or the "2-Minute Abs" or even the "1-Minute Abs?" You get the picture. It is easy to sell these contraptions, because people want the easy way out. I had the famous "Invisible Abs"—you know, the "No-See Um Abs."

I hate to break it to you, but there is no easy way out. In order to stay fit and healthy, you gotta MOVE IT! There is no such thing as "spot conditioning." Just by lying down and doing five minutes of abs on a roller or by sitting in a metal chair raising your legs up and down will not get you a terrific set of abs. In order to get great looking abs, you have to perform all-over body conditioning for your entire core muscles and eat properly. This includes full body exercise (not just abs), some cardio, and great nutrition. Underneath that layer of fat will be those strong abdominal muscles that you will work so hard to build. If you don't get rid of that layer of fat, you will never see those abdominal muscles. I know first hand; I learned by training for fitness competitions at the age of fifty!

Get Started

I don't care if you simply go outside and walk to your mailbox (if this is challenging for you): you must start somewhere. By all means, go to your doctor first and confirm you are healthy enough to begin a fitness program. If you have been cleared by your doctor to begin a fitness program, typically exercise will be the doctor's number one *prescription* for good health. This is first and foremost.

Now that step number one has been determined, let's discuss how we proceed. Realize that a fitness program must be **about you and not me** or anyone else. A great fitness program will be designed around the individual and that person's specific needs and goals. If your fitness program is designed around your specific needs, you will try hard to be successful, and you will also stay interested. The beauty of this is the program can always be changed and *should* be changed periodically.

Twenties and Thirties

When I was in my twenties and thirties, my body was completely different than in my fifties. I had so much energy and felt invincible. There wasn't anything I couldn't do; therefore, I didn't take good of care of my body as I do now. But the body is a temple, and it should be treated as such. The late night partying, eating junk food, and extracurricular activities in which you participate in your twenties and thirties will surely catch up with you in your forties and fifties and beyond.

I have always worked out in some form or fashion since my teenage years. Remember, keep it moving; I never had any money in my younger years for a health club, so I would just perform my own workout routine in my living room to music. That's OK—as long as you are doing something. Now there are all kinds of exercise DVDs to choose from if you don't want to utilize a health club or don't have the money to do so. There really is no excuse.

Pregnancy and Working Out

All you young mothers wanting to stay in shape or get into shape in your twenties and thirties: work out before your pregnancy and throughout your pregnancy *as long as your doctor says it is OK to do so*, for a healthy pregnancy and easier delivery. I worked out before I got pregnant with my first baby at seventeen years of age, and then afterwards in my living room. It was a traumatic delivery, too, considering my daughter was breech birth (sunny-side up).

With my second child eleven years later, I had joined a gym and worked out before, and was in the middle of an aerobics class when I almost passed out. That was how I knew I was pregnant. That didn't stop me. I continued to do aerobics and work out with weights throughout the entire pregnancy until I delivered my son via a natural birth in less than five hours. I bounced right back and was in my bikini within a few months.

My stomach muscles and skin were much tighter in my twenties than as a teenager. Yes, ladies, I breast-fed both of my babies, but my boobs and belly never had stretch marks or sagged. I swore by exercise and good nutrition. Remember, you can always walk in a mall or around the block. I walked daily while my dog dragged me around the block in addition to exercising.

Exercise in Your Forties

Guys and gals—get it moving if you haven't already begun an exercise program. Exercise is so important as we get older. We need to look at changing our behavior, or our muscles will begin to weaken and become stiff. This is how we get hurt with chores as simple as gardening or shopping. Don't get too caught up in losing weight, if that is your concern; instead, focus on gaining fitness. Remember that you cannot have one without the other if you want to achieve overall fitness and wellness (including your mind, body, and spirit). Balance is key.

When we are in our forties, we concentrate on so many things including our kids, households, and careers. Are you a single mom or a single dad? Then it's just that much harder—I know. When do you have time for yourself and staying fit and healthy? Well, you have to make time; if you don't do it for yourself, do it for your family. I know you are so busy, and you barely have time to come home after work, fix dinner, get kids ready for bed, and then chill for maybe thirty minutes. By then, you're just too tired—right?

Well, I know firsthand how difficult it can be, especially if you are a single parent. I used to get up fifteen minutes early in the morning and do a quick series of exercises on my living room floor while my coffee was brewing, and then go shower. Then I switched that to exercising while making dinner—in between stirring, putting food in the oven, or while something was in the skillet. Get creative.

Your body will respond beautifully in your forties if you allow it. Change the way you think about exercise and just go for it. Adults in their forties are much more serious about a fitness program than when in their twenties and thirties. We begin to realize just how important it is; we are getting that spare tire in the middle section. That literally drives me crazy. It is my worst battle and the thing I obsess over most often.

Then if the spare tire isn't enough, we get that middle-aged craze that we are "over the hill" and "no longer sexy" or "failures." Whew! Enough already. We are not over the hill, and we are sexy (it's all in our head anyway), and we aren't failing—we just simply keep trying. Change the way you are thinking. You have to appreciate who you are and what you have accomplished. If you feel you haven't done anything, then start now! Make a decision in your forties to begin a new lifestyle right now, this very minute, with a commitment while you are reading. I want you to write this down—right here—in this book so it is permanent. Write down your commitment (whatever that might be) and then just DO IT!

_____

_____

_____

_____

_____

You'll have to find the time that is right for you, your family, your lifestyle, your income level, and your schedule. By all means, make exercise a *regular part of your day*. You have to change the way of thinking about exercise. It must become a way of life for you, something that you place in your daily calendar, something that you don't think twice about—you just do it. You do it because it is good for you; it makes you feel better, stronger, and more self-confident; and it is the way to achieve your goals.

Exercise in Your Fifties

Ah, yes—the fifties. *I know who I am, and I know exactly what I want.* What a peaceful thing. You set a goal, and you do it. And my, do we set goals in our fifties! I began to think so differently about goals and fitness when I turned fifty. I knew fitness was all up to me and how I personally treated my body. When I set out to compete at fifty, trust me—that was commitment. Without an ounce of training whatsoever and no clue as to what I was doing, I had only a simple desire to do something that I'd never done before. Once I made that decision, I then set the goals and objectives to make it happen. We'll talk more about goal setting in another chapter.

Our bodies respond very differently in our fifties; I firmly believe we get stronger more easily than in our younger years. Maybe it is because we understand there is not that much time left to grab onto this wonderful thing called health and fitness and make it work for the rest of our lives. We are naturally more committed. We have to be more careful about our choice of exercise, because our bodies aren't as flexible and elastic as they were in our twenties, thirties, and forties. Knowing this makes it more important to keep exercising than ever. We have to be concerned with balance—and I'm not speaking of balance in our lives as we addressed in our twenties and thirties: I literally mean *balance*. As we grow older, we get dizzy and off-kilter. There are specific exercises to help balance.

Depending on your level of fitness at fifty, you are either continuing your journey or just beginning one. If you are just beginning, consult with your doctor for approval, and by all means start taking your *prescription* for exercise. You can work in the garden, walk the dog, build a birdhouse, or you, too, can make the decision to train for a triathlon or a fitness competition. Never say never. And never allow anyone else to set your limitations.

Exercise keeps us young—body and mind—not to mention our spirit. Let's not forget about dancing, biking, yoga, Pilates, walking or running. Exercise can reduce that stiff joint pain we feel after not moving, improve our posture, aid in circulation, and help us not be so tired. I firmly believe that fifty is the new thirty—why not make it the new twenty-five? We are only as old as we think we are anyway. I feel twenty-five; how about you?

This is very important: at fifty we naturally begin to lose our muscle tone and strength unless we build it up on purpose. Ladies, we are in danger of osteoporosis. Adding a few pounds of muscle can increase our metabolism as we age, which will help our energy level and help keep our weight intact. If we lift more weight, we are stimulating our bones to grow by placing more stress on them. Strong muscles are a significant way to help prevent bone loss. Also, having strong muscles means having safer muscles.

Our Bodies

What makes up our bodies anyway? Well, there are basically four parts: muscle mass, fat mass, water weight, and bone weight. The **muscle mass** refers to how much of our body weight is muscle. There are more than 640 skeletal muscles that control our voluntary movements. About 40 percent of our body's weight comes from the muscular system. So you see, muscle mass is very important.

The next part of our bodies is **fat mass**. Not all fat is bad and actually plays a very important part in our bodies. Fat helps to protect our internal organs and insulates the body. We learned in grammar school that the Inuits had to have extra fat to protect them against the brutal cold. Fat is important in the female reproductive system, too. We have to have a minimum level of fat to menstruate; this is why some high-power female athletes stop having periods. Fat also stores energy for us to use.

However, there is bad fat that forms easily when we become sedentary—so get moving. The bad fat is associated with diabetes and some cancers. It can negatively affect our self-esteem and unfortunately, more often than not, our sex lives. People naturally feel better about themselves when they are fit and healthy.

Our bodies are made up of more than **75 percent water**—wow! Without enough water, our digestive system and blood flow don't operate properly. This is my downfall; I don't drink enough water. We can lose up to ten cups of water throughout the day through sweating, evaporation, breathing, and waste removal. Even though our diets contain water, we will still need to drink about eight cups of water a day. Depending on your fitness level, this could even be more.

Bone weight is the percentage of bone mass in our bodies. We have 206 bones—twenty-two are located in the skull and twenty-seven are in each hand alone. Our skeletal system accounts for about 20 percent of body mass and provides a stable framework for our muscles, skin, and internal organs. Did you know that inside our bodies, our bones don't really look like they do on the CSI shows? They are actually made up of living tissue that make blood cells and store minerals like calcium. Bones are very light and yet they are five times stronger than steel. I always think about a tiny ant carrying a huge piece of food on his back and equate that to our bones being stronger than steel.

The bottom line to this discussion of what makes up our bodies is balance. We want each of these items to be in proper proportion: strong bones and muscles, relatively low percentage of body fat, and the right amount of water for our activity levels. Don't forget about how we think. Our outlook on life is very important, and balance is the key.

Flexibility is critical for any age; however, it is even more important as we age. We have all seen people as they age and develop a "stooped over" posture, so please sit up straight and carry yourself strong with your shoulders back. Flexibility decreases as we age just like our bone density. It is so important to stretch and then stretch again. Do very light stretching before you exercise, because you can pull a muscle. It is far more important to stretch very well after you work out so you are stretching warm muscles and thereby decreasing your chances of pulling one.

It seems like I have had a pulled groin muscle since my early twenties that hasn't fully gotten well. I remember the very minute I did it, too. I was participating in a Kenpo Karate class and stretching, and the instructor said go down further and then further. I felt it basically rip. To this day, my left groin muscle on the inside of my leg hurts if I stretch too far or move the wrong way. So I am very careful how I stretch. This can become very difficult when you are fifty and competing in fitness competitions!

Benefits of Exercise

When you have been sitting for a long time and then get up and walk very quickly across a room, have you experienced how your heart begins to race just a bit? Your body knows it is doing a form of exercise and is telling your blood flow to pick up, which gets your heart pumping to handle the action. We use two forms of exercise: aerobic and anaerobic.

Aerobic means "with oxygen." This takes me back to the Jane Fonda days with the leggings wrapped all the way up to my thighs and my body suit with the T-back and tights underneath. Don't forget about the matching headband. Now think about stepping up and down on a bench—boot camps, low-impact aerobics, dance, walking and running—and you get the idea of aerobic exercise. When blood delivers oxygen to our cells to meet this need to produce energy, then our aerobic system is the dominant method of producing energy.

Anaerobic, on the flip side, anaerobic means without oxygen. When a muscle must lift a heavy weight quickly, it will depend upon our anaerobic methods for producing energy. We really can't use our anaerobic methods to produce energy for very long. We can use anaerobic methods for performing sprints, but for long-term exercising, we use the aerobic system for sustaining energy. The more we exercise aerobically over a period of time, the more we get used to it, and so does our cardiovascular system. This means it gets easier, and we have to ramp it up by increasing intensity. This helps make our hearts healthier.

Interval Training

Interval training is one of my favorite forms of training. It is also an excellent way to start out if you are new to aerobic fitness. This form of exercising can be as easy as running fast for a sprint, then slow jogging or walking, and then starting over. It can be stair climbing followed by walking in place. You don't have to be a highly trained athlete to perform interval training. Intervals should last between one and two minutes of vigorous exercise, like sprints or jumping rope, followed by rest intervals of walking or a slower-paced exercise. You can repeat these steps anywhere from five to ten times depending upon your fitness level and goals.

I used to participate in a form of boot camp training in my mid-forties, and I absolutely loved it. The instructor pushed a group of exercisers, and I pushed myself. Over a period of a year, I realized that I was capable of anything that I set my mind to. When I first started out, I thought I was going to die of a heart attack—no kidding. Then I kept repeating to myself, "I can do this, I can do this." And I did. Today, I make up my own interval training routine with running sprints forward and then running backwards, running sideways like football players do, and jumping rope. I'll even add in twenty minutes of kickboxing before I hit the treadmill for power walking. So you see, it doesn't have to be in a class setting; you can make up your own. Just remember—keep moving.

Weight Training

Guys and gals, you gotta do this. Ladies, you will not build huge muscles like the guys will, so that cannot be used as an excuse. What you will do is to build muscles to help protect your bones, tone your bodies, build self-confidence, and look better in your clothes.

Guys, I really don't have to tell you what it will do, but why not? You will develop a better muscular frame, become stronger, increase your strength, and also increase your libido. This last point should be enough to begin your push-ups today. The specific reps and loads will be determined based on your individual goals. If you can afford it, then it would be advisable to locate a qualified, certified fitness trainer who will develop a program around your specific needs and goals—not theirs.

You will begin to see results in as little as a week if you are beginning a new program. You'll notice that your muscles will become sore after a good workout at two different times. The first time is during or immediately after exercising. This is from lactic acid buildup in the muscles, which irritates the nerve endings. After an hour or so, the bloodstream will begin to remove most of this lactic acid. This is also why it is critical to cool down (stretch) after exercising. Keeping your blood flowing allows these waste products to be carried away more quickly. Generally, my second day is the worst; I get very stiff; this is the second type of soreness. This may continue into a third day depending upon the intensity of the workout. There are minor tears in the connective tissues that hold the muscle fibers together and in the muscle cell membranes, and these cause soreness. It is weird to think that we actually have to tear our muscles for them to get stronger and more toned. Keep in mind that this is different than actually tearing a muscle or pulling a muscle to the point that it is an injury. Minor tears caused by a designed workout actually build muscle. Remember, stretch warm muscles, not cold ones, and drink lots of water. Massage will also help get rid of waste products, too. You should also consider eating a banana if you are low in potassium, which can also cause soreness. As you keep exercising, you will become more fit and the soreness will decrease or diminish.

Start your Exercise Program Today—Exercise Is for Any Age

I think we've spent enough time together now that you will trust me when I say, "Exercise is for any age." It's not just for the young or a specific age group or gender; it is for every single one of us. We must get moving and keep it moving in order to lead healthy, productive, and active lives. Exercise will help us maintain balance—not only in mind, body, and spirit, but literally our balance, so we don't fall as we get older. Please make an appointment with your doctor today if you are new to exercising and request your *prescription* for exercise. Tell your doctor—"Sharon sent me!"

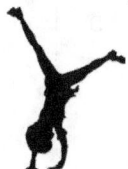

Nutrition Made Easy

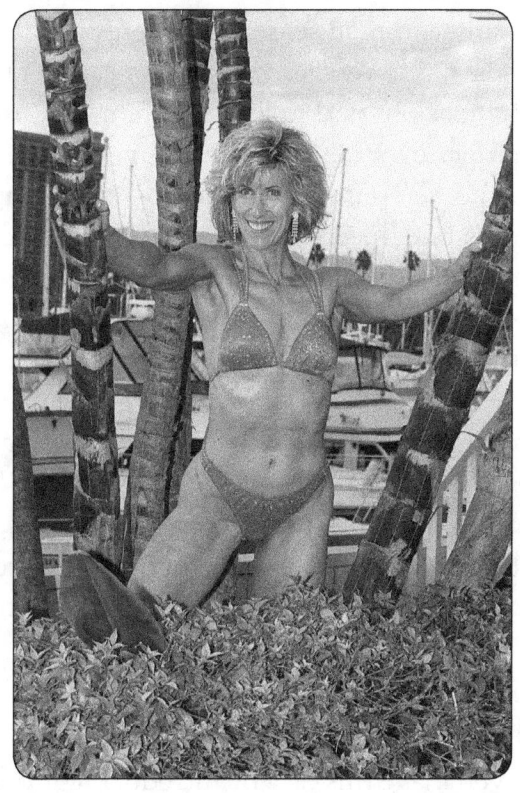

What is it that everyone wants to hear? "Nutrition is easy!" Well, it is. I have a secret that I will share with you. The key to a good nutrition plan is *non-processed food and small, frequent meals*. If you can stick to these two things, you've got it made.

OK—what is a *non-processed food*? This plentiful list includes various forms of seafood (swimmers), foul (fliers), potatoes and vegetables (things that come out of the ground), and fruits and nuts (things that fall out of trees)—and of course, oatmeal. This list is certainly not complete, but it will give you an idea of how easy it is to begin your new nutritional plan.

Energy Source

Food is energy, so you will need to choose wisely for the activities you want to be successful with while maintaining an appropriate weight for your body's composition. This is really not an exact science; it is mainly common sense. The energy going into the body includes the foods and beverages you consume, and the energy leaving the body includes physical activity, excrements (urine and feces), and your body functions (i.e. breathing, digestion, brain and heart function, blood and nervous system function, and temperature regulation). The body's basic needs use about 60 percent of your energy, physical activity will take about 30 percent, and the remaining 10 percent will be used in digestion of food and nutrient absorption.

There are other factors contributing to the way we use our energy. Age and genetics will have an effect; also gender, height, weight, body composition, diet history, and the amount of physical activity we utilize. *In order to lose it, you've got to move it.* You will have to consider if you want to run a marathon, lose baby weight, ride bicycles, work out in the gym, or simply be able to play with your grandchildren. For some people, it will be an accomplishment to walk around the block.

Powerhouse Foods

Let me help you make this easy by introducing my favorite powerhouse foods. By eating a variety of these food groups, you will have a jump start towards a good nutrition plan, more energy, weight management, and good health. Let's look at each group individually.

Blueberries—absolutely my favorite fruit! This little powerhouse berry was ranked number one in the antioxidant category by the U.S. Department of Agriculture when compared to forty other common fruits and vegetables. The benefits from the antioxidants in blueberries include protection from premature aging and better skin tone; research has also shown antioxidants in blueberries can help ward off certain types of cancer. Toss a handful into your oatmeal, low-fat yogurt, fruit smoothie, or cereal every morning. I have added them to whole grain waffles and pancakes; I even toss them over my salads. Don't forget the blueberry's sister, the blackberry. You can do the exact same thing with blackberries, which are incredible when they are in season. My husband is convinced eating blueberries is why my skin has stayed so young for over fifty years.

Wild Salmon—not the farm-raised type—is one of the best foods available for omega-3 fatty acids, which will keep your skin beautiful, supple, and moisturized— *youthful*. Salmon has selenium in it, which is a mineral that protects your skin from sun exposure. Selenium also aids in boosting our mood. The vitamin D in salmon helps keep our bones and teeth strong, too. The most recent research shows the best way to get vitamin D is a few minutes in natural sunshine daily; but be very careful with this—just a few minutes in the sun without protection. There are lots of ways to add this powerhouse food to your regular nutrition plan, so you shouldn't have any trouble. Try grilling the salmon, baking it, adding it to pasta, topping a salad with it, in sushi, or as a main course with a side of asparagus and sweet potato.

Sweet Potato—a perfect time to discuss my favorite carbohydrate; yes, it is included in the family of complex carbohydrates. I added this wonderful powerhouse food to my daily nutrition plan when I discovered its health and antiaging benefits during training for competition, but the sweet potato is a little hidden treasure that should be eaten more often than not during competition training—or at Thanksgiving covered with marshmallows. Sweet potatoes are loaded with beta-carotene, an antioxidant that fights *aging*. How cool is that? Beta-carotene is also beneficial in protecting our eyesight. I have learned to love my sweet potato just plain as a side with my dinner, but you can mash them or cut them up and bake as a form of healthy "French fry." If you do this, try sprinkling just a bit of cinnamon on them, which also has health benefits. You can also serve them cut, roasted, and tossed with herbs and onions as an awesome side if your taste buds require seasoning. You can even make sweet potato soup or sweet potato spinach salad.

Spinach—I used to watch *Popeye the Sailor Man*—with his large bicep and girlfriend with the skinny legs—when I was a kid. Well, Popeye was certainly onto something with this leafy green powerhouse vegetable rich in nutrients and antioxidants. Spinach is just loaded with lutein, which keeps your eyesight healthy. Spinach is also a wonderful source of vitamins B, C, E, potassium, calcium, iron, magnesium, and omega-3 fatty acids. I think you can begin to see a pattern with the powerhouse foods. I like to top my romaine salads with spinach leaves or simply make a large spinach salad to stand on its own. You can also sauté spinach either plain or with mushrooms and red onions for a quick, healthy side. Some of the pizza restaurants are catching on to the amazing health benefits of spinach and adding spinach to pizzas and pastas with tomatoes.

Tomatoes—I have to absolutely have these little powerhouse morsels everyday. I add them to salads, eat them as a breakfast side, or I simply just add cherry tomatoes as a side for tuna (chunk light variety). Tomatoes are the best source of the antiaging antioxidant lycopene, which is more easily absorbed by your body when it is cooked or processed. You can get this form of tomatoes in canned tomato sauce, tomato juice, and ketchup. Regarding these cooked versions, however, you will have to be careful and consult with your doctor if you are watching your sodium and sugar intake.

Walnuts—Love them; gotta have them! You don't have to eat huge amounts of walnuts to enjoy the health benefits including smoother skin, shinier hair, brighter eyes, and stronger bones. I get my daily dose of nutrients like omega-3 fatty acids and vitamin E by simply tossing a small handful on top of my oatmeal each morning. You can also add them to your salad, pasta, spinach salad, or dessert.

Yogurt—Women and children need calcium. One cup of low-fat yogurt has more calcium than a cup of fat-free milk, and adding yogurt is sometimes more convenient than adding milk to a nutrition plan. Yogurt is great for our posture, nails, and teeth. You can mix it with fruit and granola for a healthy breakfast or snack or add it in a smoothie shake for an added benefit. One of my dessert recipes includes one layer of blueberries or blackberries, one layer of bananas, one layer of yogurt, and a sprinkle of walnuts and chips of dark chocolate on top. For the kids, sprinkle just a little bit of Cheerios over the top for added fun.

Dark Chocolate—Oh my goodness! Did we just add dark chocolate to our list of powerhouse foods? Am I your girlfriend now? I cannot give up my chocolate, and I was totally beside myself when research proved that dark chocolate has health benefits. Dark chocolate helps skin stay hydrated and protected from sun damage. Research has also shown, contrary to popular belief, that chocolate does not cause acne. Before you run out and buy the expensive dark chocolates, keep in mind the best kind of chocolate has a high flavanol content and should be at least 60 percent cacao. Hershey's has a wonderful dark chocolate that meets both the budget and the health benefit criteria. I don't think I need to tell you how to add chocolate to your diet; do as I do—PUT IT ON EVERYTHING!

Kiwis—What a funny looking fruit! This small, fuzzy brown oval is loaded with vitamin C and antioxidants. Remember that antioxidants and vitamin C keep the skin firm, help prevent wrinkles, and are great for healthy bones and teeth. There are many cosmetics now made with vitamin C for the reasons we are discussing. The antioxidants in kiwis are also known to protect you from certain types of cancer and heart disease. So eat up these little fruits that are just plain ugly on the outside and simply beautiful and scrumptious on the inside. You can also use them as a garnish for most dishes and then eat the slices.

Oysters—I have to mention this mysterious seafood in my powerhouse food based on a terrible childhood memory. At my junior high prom, I went to dinner with friends who dared me to chew up this slimy little creature—and I did. I don't typically partake in this little mystery, but a lot of other people do. Oysters are a good source of zinc, which aids in skin cell renewal and repair. Zinc also keeps your nails, hair, and eyes healthy. Oysters have also been touted as an aphrodisiac, but I cannot attest to this theory. Who cares, anyway—if you look and feel beautiful, you won't require an aphrodisiac.

Small Meals

Now you have the basics for a great nutrition plan to live by, so let's discuss how to include them within your daily routine. The second part of my secret is to eat small meals throughout the day. For example, a small meal might include a piece of fish or poultry equal to a size of a deck of cards, and a one-ounce snack could equal the size of a container of Altoids. I use the rule of thumb that my portion of veggies should be double in size to my fish or poultry. Sometimes I will split my evening sweet potato and add it to my next day snack of chicken breast bites.

Keep in mind: I did not say to *diet*. The first three letters in the word *diet* are D.I.E. If we can transition from this line of thinking to become more nutritionally conscious and to develop a way to live our lives for longevity and not for the moment, then we understand the second part of the secret: small, healthy meals. There are three nutrients that provide our bodies with the energy it needs, and they are called macronutrients: carbohydrates, protein, and fat.

Carbohydrates (Carbs)—Carbs are a necessary component to your nutrition plan. Carbs provide us with our thinking capability and energy; in fact, carbs are our primary energy source. They give direct energy to our brain for the thinking component, direct energy to our central nervous system, and direct energy to our muscles by using protein to build and repair muscle tissue and cells. There are three main types of carbs we can consume: simple sugars, complex carbs, and dietary fiber. The simple sugars require little or no digestion for us to utilize them. They give us quick bursts of energy and unfortunately are followed by a drop in blood sugar and energy level. You can find simple sugars in fruit and fruit juices, candy, soft drinks, and sweeteners including corn syrup, honey, and table sugars.

In contrast to simple sugars, complex carbs provide our bodies with a more sustained energy source. Complex carbs can be grouped as fresh vegetables and fruits, beans, and natural whole grains. For the most benefit, the main focus should be on whole grain sources of complex carbs including oatmeal, whole grain breads, and Cheerios. Whole grain complex carbs are broken down and released into the bloodstream more slowly than the simple sugars. They keep blood sugar more even and help us feel satisfied for longer periods of time. For even more energy, try high fiber and low glycemic foods such as brown rice, barley, sweet potatoes, buckwheat, pumpernickel bread, skim milk, nonfat/no-sugar-added milk, beans and legumes, apples, berries (dark is great for you), cherries, pears, kiwi, and non-starchy vegetables. This last group includes broccoli, which is absolutely the best vegetable choice you can make. Also included within this list are asparagus, carrots, spinach, cauliflower, zucchini, peppers, summer squash, mushrooms, and leafy green vegetables. As you can see, the list offers quite a variety of choices.

Our last carbohydrate to review is very important for our bodies: dietary fiber. The recommended daily serving of dietary fiber is twenty to thirty grams, which can be found in bran cereal, avocados, legumes and beans (including pinto beans and black beans). Americans get plenty of simple sugars and refined carbs in our diets but consume much less fiber. We need fiber for healthy digestion to help us to feel full, keep us regular, and also aid in preventing some diseases. Carbs have received a bad reputation in recent years due to low-carb fad diets. However, eating carbs supplies our bodies with necessary energy and nutrients while serving so many other purposes. The important thing to remember when choosing carbs is to pick whole grains instead of refined starches and to eat foods that are good sources of dietary fiber. Exercising without eating carbs is like driving a car without gas. The body will find it very difficult to perform without its main source of energy.

Protein—We have to have protein; it is the body's major building material. This necessary component makes up the brain, muscles, blood, skin, hair, nails, and connective tissue. Protein aids in tissue growth and maintenance, and helps keep us strong. It makes enzymes and some hormones that regulate body processes, and provides antibodies for our immune system. Amino acids are the building blocks of protein; substances, both essential and nonessential, that make up protein. We need to ingest enough essential amino acids each day to provide our bodies with an adequate source of protein.

Good sources of protein include lean cuts of meats, peanut butter (natural is preferred, or almond butter), beans, milk, cheese, poultry, soy products, yogurt, eggs, fish, legumes, and nuts. When consuming an incomplete protein (found in plant products) like rice or beans, combine with another protein to provide all the essential amino acids needed by our bodies—rice *and* beans. Food combining allows vegetarians to provide their bodies with the necessary essential components of protein. Be conscious in preparation to trim visible fat from meat, and bake, broil, boil, grill, or roast instead of frying. Chunk light tuna also provides a good source of protein and can be purchased in very convenient packages perfect for lunch or traveling. I typically carry one with me in my purse when I have to travel, and it is accepted onboard airlines. And remember, when we exercise, we break down muscle tissue. Protein is needed to help rebuild muscle fibers following workouts. Food sources of protein also provide several other essential nutrients including zinc, iron, and Vitamin B-12.

Fat— You have to have fat in your nutrition plan. Yes, I said FAT! Good fat, that is, not the kind I sneak and eat while watching my favorite television show. Fat provides a ready source of energy and fatty acids necessary for chemical activities. They carry fat-soluble vitamins (A, D, E, K) and increase satiety with food. Fat certainly makes eating more enjoyable and aids in temperature regulation. It is an extremely concentrated energy source, which is great for endurance activities. Fat remains in our stomach longer than carbs or protein, helping us feel full longer. It is needed to carry essential fatty acids throughout our bodies, and essential fatty acids are needed to produce certain hormones and must be provided by a person's diet. Types of fat include omega-3, omega-6, monounsaturated, saturated, and trans fat.

The omega-3 and omega-6 fats are types of polyunsaturated fats and are essential for building a strong immune system and healthy skin. Remember I mentioned earlier that we are setting a pattern with non-processed foods providing us with youthful skin? Omega-3s also protect our heart, as well as protecting us from some cancers, immune disorders, and arthritis. Good sources are salmon, flaxseed meal and oil, nuts, soybeans, and canola oils. Omega-6s keep our skin and brain functioning healthy. People need less of these omegas since our diets supply them readily. Some sources of omega-6 include corn, sunflower, and other vegetable oils.

The heart-healthy fats are monounsaturated and can be found in canola oil, olive oil, peanuts, avocados, and olives. They help decrease total cholesterol levels, decrease LDL cholesterol levels, and may contribute to increasing HDL cholesterol levels. I personally know this to be a fact. When I am in training for a competition and am really watching my "bad fat" intake, leaving behind the good fats, my cholesterol levels drop by as much as 10 percent. During my off-season, they actually go back up because I am not as conscious of my bad fat intake.

When purchasing foods, read the labels and notice the amount of *saturated fats and trans fatty acids* (hydrogenated fats) in the ingredients. Saturated fats increase cholesterol levels thus increasing risk for heart disease. This fat is found in butter, margarine, fatty meats, full-fat dairy products, and most fast foods. Trans fat is formed when vegetable oils are hydrogenated, and they are as harmful as saturated for your heart health. They can be found in most baked goods, crackers, chips, margarine, and fast foods because it extends the shelf life of many food products. Trans fat offers no nutritional value.

What's in a label? The FDA did not begin regulating food labels until 1994. Now our labels contain information like percent daily value, fats (good and bad), trans fats, cholesterol, fiber, sugar, calories from fat, serving size, and if the food claims to be light or low fat. Pay attention to the first ingredient on the label, which is typically the most prominent. If "partially hydrogenated" (or hydrogenated oil) is listed on the ingredient list in the first five items, then the product is high in trans fat and should be avoided. Trans fat can be found in most baked goods, and it extends the shelf life of many food products. Choose *fresh, non-processed over processed or "pre-packaged" items.* Some of these trans fatty foods include traditional peanut butter (read the labels to find one that does not include trans fats), packaged apple pies, glazed donuts, vegetable shortening, wheat thins, pot pies, cookies, some corn chips, and muffin and pancake mixes. Again, read the labels. Some of the manufacturers are catching on, and they are making a conscious effort to become healthier with the 2006 FDA regulation requiring them to state the grams of trans fatty acids in a product.

Fluids—Next on our list are fluids, which are important in keeping our bodies properly hydrated. I will not try and administer a proper dosage of fluids for your specific body composition. If you need this, you may consult with a doctor. I have to admit right now that I do not drink enough water, and my body suffers from it. What I will tell you is we have to consume fluids to perspire, urinate and defecate, and breathe.

The primary function of water in our body is to regulate every living cell's processes and chemical reactions. Fluids help form protein and glycogen in our bodies, and act as solvent for minerals, vitamins, and other nutrients. They play a key role in the digestion, absorption, transportation, and use of food nutrients. Fluids help excrete waste products and toxins, thus eliminating constipation. Stop right here—I need to clarify that I do not believe in or endorse colon-cleansing products. Eating a good nutritional plan with plenty of fluids will provide the same health benefits and save unnecessary wear and tear on your organs. Fluids aid in new tissue development and help maintain proper body temperature. They also provide a protective cushion for tissue by lubricating joints.

You may be able to tell if you are not consuming enough fluids by the look of your skin, stiff joints, dry skin, or constipation. But what if you are getting plenty of fluids; can you still get dehydrated? Absolutely, you can. When you consume the majority of your fluids in the form of caffeine or alcohol, are exposed to heavy heat, use diuretics or laxatives, exercise excessively, or deplete your carbohydrate intake, you will be in danger of dehydration. Consult your doctor for specifics on fluid intake for your goals and activity level.

Weight Management

Remember our discussion of consuming small meals throughout the day. The traditional thinking has always been to eat three meals a day with the last meal being the largest. Let's change this theory completely to begin your day with a wonderful breakfast, complete with a complex carb, fruit, protein, and a good fat. You may accomplish this with a simple bowl of oatmeal, blueberries, walnuts, egg whites, and a side of English muffin or wheat muffin. This will help with your cognitive thinking for the rest of the day. Also, because you know you consumed a healthy breakfast, you will instinctively want to eat well the rest of the day.

Eat three main meals a day with two small meals (healthy snacks), and use smaller plates. Remember to eat a protein, a complex carb (from our list if necessary), vegetables, and a healthy fat. Store food out of sight, and keep healthy snacks on hand with tempting foods out of the house. Practice portion control, and limit refined sugars and excess fat consumption (especially the bad fat). Drink plenty of water, and eat a piece of fruit in lieu of a glass of juice. Use low-fat cooking methods such as baking, grilling, roasting, and broiling. Also, limit sugar and alcohol intake. Eating foods low in saturated fat and trans fat is the most effective dietary way to lower blood cholesterol levels as well as lose weight. At least 50 percent of your meal should come from a wide variety of fruits and vegetables (preferably fresh). Canned varieties generally harbor added salt and sugar.

For weight loss, the National Institutes of Health recommend a 10 percent reduction over six months for optimal weight maintenance. A healthy weight-loss goal is half a pound to two pounds per week. More than that will surely result in regaining the weight. The basic formula for weight loss is "Eat fewer calories + Exercise more = Weight loss + Better health." It is not about how much weight you lose; it is more important how you feel about yourself and whether you have a healthy body composition. The key to any successful weight-loss program is to take in fewer calories than are expended through the calorie-burning process. Therefore, exercise is always an important part of any weight-loss program. Most people gain weight slowly as a result of consuming slightly more calories than they are able to take off each day.

When I turned fifty, I was not involved in as many physical activities as I was in my twenties, so gaining weight was easier. If you take in just fifty calories more than your body can use each day, then you can expect to gain approximately five pounds during the course of a year. This information is available throughout Internet research Web sites including *How Dieting Works, The President's Council on Physical Fitness and Sports,* and *Organic Food Bar.*

Healthy Tips

Choose fats wisely, get your omega-3 fatty acids, limit salt and sugar intake, drink plenty of liquids, and eat a better breakfast for a perfect start to the day. Make sure your nutritional plan includes plenty of fresh fruits and vegetables and is low in total fat and saturated fat. The majority of your eating plan should be from plant sources including fruits and vegetables, potatoes, breads and grains, beans, nuts, and seeds, olive oil being the principal fat and used in lieu of other fats such as butter or margarine. You should keep your daily consumption of low to moderate amounts of nonfat milk and yogurt, and low-fat cheese; fish and chicken weekly or throughout the week (depending on your choice of protein); and lean red meat only once or twice a month (unless you are in competition or advised by your doctor).

Sample Meals: Breakfast. We have already looked at a healthy breakfast with oatmeal. For added benefits of oatmeal, use the steel-cut version found at health food stores. The steel-cut oats take longer to cook, contain more cholesterol lowering fiber and take longer to digest, so they help you feel fuller longer and are basically less processed. I use the weight control packaged version for convenience and time. You can top with wheat germ, ground flax seed, raisins, cinnamon, blueberries, blackberries, bananas, and walnuts.

If oatmeal is not your thing, try layering three cups of nonfat plain yogurt, twelve ounces of unsweetened fruit such as fresh or frozen berries and melon, and eight tablespoons of low-fat granola (makes four servings). You can also do something similar with a fruit smoothie and add your favorite protein powder; I only recommend one shake a day if you utilize protein powder. Remember to keep everything as natural as possible, utilizing non-processed forms of food sources.

One of my most requested breakfast recipes is the *Powerhouse Pancakes*, with just 281 calories, 16% fat (5 g; 0 g sat), 34% carbs (24 g), 50% protein (35 g), 5 g fiber, 40 mg calcium, 2 mg iron, and 114 mg sodium. The recipe serves four and requires less than ten minutes for prep time and cooking.

2 cups cooked steel-cut oatmeal

8 egg whites

2 cups water

1 teaspoon cinnamon

4 scoops vanilla whey protein powder (brand is your choice)

Nonfat cooking spray

1 cup sliced fresh strawberries (or other berries of your choice)

4 tablespoons nonfat plain yogurt (optional)

In a large bowl, combine the oatmeal, egg whites, water, cinnamon, and protein powder. Coat a medium nonstick skillet with cooking spray, and heat on medium-high. Place two heaping tablespoons of batter on the skillet. Cook three minutes or until they are dry around the edges. Turn and cook the other side until golden brown. Top with yogurt, if desired, and strawberries.

Eggs and toast: Prepare two omega-3 enriched eggs, any style, using two teaspoons of trans-fat-free margarine. Serve eggs with one slice of whole-wheat toast with two teaspoons of fruit spread. (If you poach or boil the eggs, use the margarine on your bread). I like mine without any margarine. Serve with 3/4 cup of raspberries or strawberries, fresh or thawed from frozen, and one cup of skim milk.

Lunch. My all-time favorite lunch is a large, green, leafy salad topped with spinach leaves, carrots, tomatoes, small orange slices, a teaspoon of almond oil, and a 2.6 ounce package of chunk light tuna (18 grams protein). I have a large Wasa cracker on the side to watch calories and get my carbs. You can add a banana with a small amount of natural peanut butter or almond butter as a snack.

Tuna pita: Stuff a six-inch, whole-wheat pita with green, leafy lettuce or spinach and a five-ounce (one bowl) package of flavored tuna (your choice). Serve with one cup of carrot sticks and twenty calories' worth of dressing or almond oil.

On-the-go lunch: One-part-skim mozzarella cheese stick, one large apple, and 1/3 a cup of almonds; or a sub sandwich made with whole-wheat bread, lettuce, tomatoes, and vegetables of your choice.

Dinner. Depending on your schedule, dinner can be as simple as pasta with shrimp and veggies or grilled salmon with one cup of cooked wild rice and veggies, or, if time permits, you could try this wonderful dish with either cod or salmon. This recipe serves four and will provide 282 calories, 32 g protein, 23 g carbs, 7 g fat, 2 g sat fat, 3 g mono fat, 74 mg cholesterol, 0 g fiber, 550 g sodium. Be sure to add vegetables like broccoli and a sweet potato for your fiber needs.

Canola oil spray

1/2 cup orange juice

2 tablespoons honey

1 clove garlic, minced

1½ pounds cod or salmon fillets

1/2 teaspoon cornstarch

1 orange, peeled and sliced in rings

Preheat the oven to 350 degrees. Spray an ovenproof dish with nonfat cooking spray. In a bowl, mix together orange juice, honey, and garlic. Place fillets in the dish and cover with the orange juice mixture. Place the dish on the top shelf in the oven and bake for ten to twelve minutes, depending on thickness. Remove fish to serving plates. Add cornstarch to remaining orange sauce in a saucepan. Cook and stir frequently on the stovetop on a low temperature until thickened. Pour over the fish and garnish with orange slices.

For more healthy tips and recipes, you can visit my Web site at www.FitnessAnyAge.com. When I am in training for competition, my nutrition plan becomes a lot more rigid and, quite frankly, boring! We'll discuss the competition plan in another chapter. For now, let's enjoy the fruits of our labor and eat very healthily so we can enjoy a beautiful piece of dark chocolate.

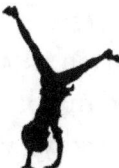

Supplements/Drugs—
To Do or Not to Do

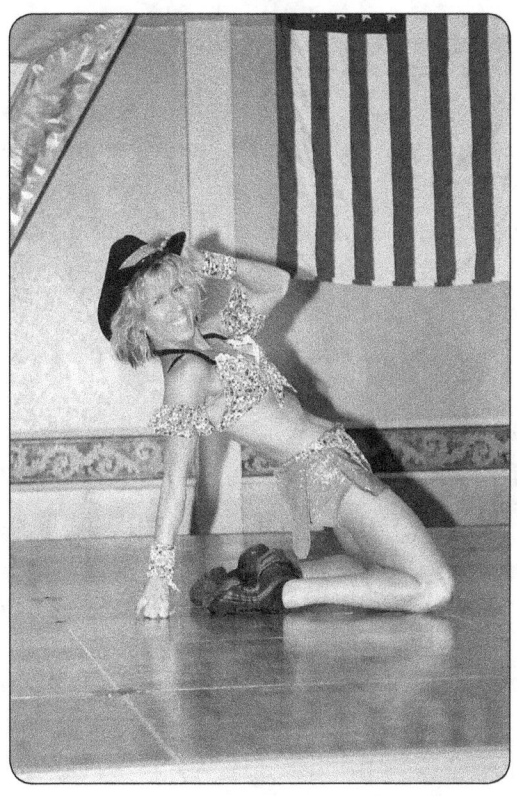

This chapter will be very delicate because of the controversy surrounding the subject. I have never—repeat, never—utilized supplements or drugs in training for any of my fitness shows, nor do I use them in my everyday life. Putting it plain and simple: you don't need them! Oh sure, they definitely do give you the edge you need in competition, but you must ask yourself, "Are the long-term effects really worth it?" That is a personal question, and one that I cannot answer for you; for me, there's no question about it. I don't do it.

It is a fact that you will see my picture on several of the supplement Web sites, which would lead you to believe that I have participated in supplementation. Quite the contrary; when a person signs the release to appear in a major fitness show, there is a clause stating that you agree to their use of your picture in advertising. So there you go; it looks like I am advertising for their product even though I have never tried it.

Vitamins

Most of us cannot possibly get all the nutrients our body requires on a daily basis, so a daily multivitamin may be essential for you. You should always consult your doctor before taking any kind of vitamin, supplement, or any other drug. Certain vitamins can interfere with other medications, and some supplements can be detrimental to your health when mixed with medications. So I remind you again to consult with your doctor.

During my research, I discovered that even multivitamins have been associated with greater breast density in premenopausal women, which could be associated with cancer. This report was published in the May 2008 issue of the *American Journal of Clinical Nutrition.* The report doesn't say that women taking multivitamins should stop taking them, but they should consult with their doctors to be aware of the associated risks. The report also recommends women with dense breasts to have regular mammograms and possibly additional ultrasounds.

There are some vitamins that have proven to be beneficial, such as B-12 supplements for the elderly population and folic acid for women of childbearing age. I take calcium with added vitamin D, because my doctor ordered me to do so after I turned fifty to help protect my bone health. For most people, the micronutrients we get from our food will generally be enough to protect us against any vitamin deficiencies, which are rare in the U.S.

Most people take their vitamins like they are some sort of candy, thinking that vitamins will save them and make them healthy—not the case, ladies and gentlemen. You have to get proper nutrition to remain healthy. I used to work with a woman who told me a story about a friend of hers who was diagnosed with leukemia. His family was devastated, and the doctors were trying everything to help him. One of the doctors asked the man to bring in every single supplement and vitamin he was taking on his next doctor visit. The man brought in what appeared to be a suitcase filled with all kinds of vitamins and supplements; his doctor ordered him to STOP taking everything immediately. Miraculously, the man's symptoms went away, and his follow-up blood tests proved that all indications for leukemia had vanished. The man never had leukemia; he was basically killing himself with vitamins and supplements.

Again, I want to stress: do whatever your doctor has recommended for your nutritional and health needs. What is good for one person may not be the right thing for another individual.

L-Glutamine and Other Supplements

I have researched this supplement because I've heard so much about the benefits, and there are both good and bad references. I have to admit the benefits that people claim are very enticing. On the other hand, research has proven enough for me to stay away from taking an L-Glutamine supplement—especially at my age. I would absolutely only take this supplement under strict orders from my doctor and only in certain instances (i.e., stomach disorders, chemotherapy). I would challenge you to do as I have done and research this supplement on your own. I really do not want to provide too much information, because the research is so varied and contradictory. Pay little attention to the bodybuilding Web sites, as they are not going to provide the hard-core medical research that you need in order to make an intelligent decision based on facts. The reason I mention this particular supplement is that it is discussed as a miracle drug on most sites—be aware.

Caffeine and Precursor Testosterone

As I mentioned at the beginning of the chapter, this is a very delicate subject because I am sure I am stepping on some toes; but tiptoe I must. If you choose to participate in supplement and drug use for whatever reason, then by all means know the dangers and what will possibly happen to you in future years. Don't kid yourself when reading the ingredients (please read and research); most of the drugs and supplements are filled with caffeine and serve as a precursor testosterone. Caffeine abuse symptoms can include sleeplessness, tremors, nausea, vomiting, chest pains, and heart palpitations, among others. Some of the products that contain harmful levels of caffeine have been removed from the store shelves. The use of precursor testosterones and/or pro-hormones may result in dangerous side effects similar to those that steroids produce including an increase in estrogen, hair loss, benign prostate enlargement, and acne. Do you really need this stuff? What are your goals—to look good for the moment or live a long healthy life?

Closing Statement

So there is no mistake about how I feel regarding the subject of supplements and drug use, let me say it again: I don't believe in it and do not participate in it. I have never looked or felt as good as I do right now in my fifties, and one of the reasons is that I have never made use of supplements and drugs other than what my doctor recommends. You will find a wide use of drugs and supplements in both the bodybuilding world and the fitness world. I don't care what they say—they do it! It's not hearsay; I've seen it. Bottom line is, you will have to make your own choice, one that is good for your own health and well being in alignment with your goals.

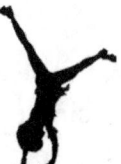

Setting Goals—The Process

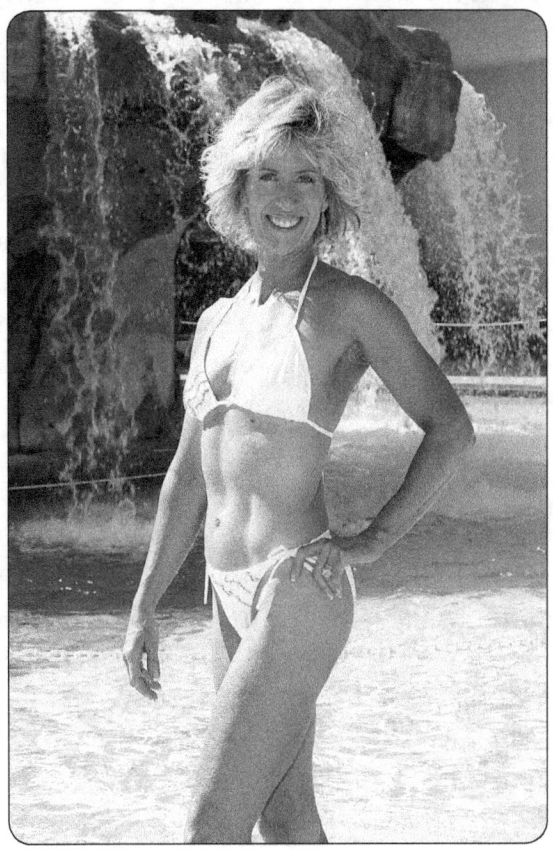

OK—so you've read about nutrition, exercise, and supplements. Now what do you do? I'll break it down step-by-step and make it very easy for you to establish a plan to meet your goals and objectives for a healthier you. We will talk about a *small wins strategy* and *goal setting*. I can help you do this; all I ask from you is that you open your mind to what we are discussing and *believe in yourself.* The reason I ask you to do this part is because I can't do it for you.

Small Wins Strategy

I studied the *small wins strategy* years ago in school. Basically, we will do a little something every single day to meet our goal. It could be something as small as looking something up on the Internet referencing a healthy food to see the amount of vitamin content. The effort involved is a step toward meeting your goal for nutrition and exercise. So we will reward you, in our theory of a *small wins strategy*. It is based on dividing up a larger problem into limited units that can be attacked individually. You will feel empowered when you celebrate small wins towards the larger goal.

A small win could be something as easy as adding one more repetition to your basic workout plan which would add more challenge. It could be making a decision to walk just two more houses around the block or to stop smoking by decreasing by one cigarette a day. Do you get the gist? Always reward yourself for every single small win you achieve—no matter how small or insignificant it may seem. It is an accomplishment towards your goal; therefore, it is a *small win*.

Goal Setting

Just like the *small wins strategy*, I also studied *goal setting* with each of my degree programs; especially in the master's concentration in human resource management (MAOM), you must understand the basics of how to set a goal. A lot of people have had success with the theory of *SMART Goals*, written by E. A. Locke and G. P. Latham in 1990. Let's break down SMART step by step:

S –   The goal must be **specific.** That is why our next section asks you in Step One to determine specifically what you want to accomplish and then set specific goals; clearly identify the goal: for example, losing ten pounds.

M –   The goal must be **measurable.** This takes goals beyond specific: for example, instead of losing ten pounds, lose one to two pounds a week. This is what makes this goal *measurable*. If you lose one to two pounds a week, you can measure your progress towards your main goal of losing ten pounds.

Do you get it? You have to be able to evaluate the accomplishment of a measurable goal.

A – Is your goal **aligned** with your overall purpose? Will the accomplishment of this goal contribute to the overall good? In our example, will losing one to two pounds a week contribute to your main goal of losing ten pounds overall? Sure it will.

R – Is your goal **reachable?** You have to ask yourself, Is this goal **realistic**? Is this specific goal within my capacity to achieve? This does not mean you get off the hook, either, or that your goal must be easy. Reachable does not mean that it is easily achieved. Research from Locke & Latham indicates that a more difficult goal (i.e. a *stretch goal*) is a better motivator of behavior and results in overall higher levels of accomplishment than an easy goal.

T – Setting a **time** for accomplishing your goal is critical to success. If your goal had no ending point, then it would not be effective when a deadline for accomplishment is not clear. That is why we said losing one to two pounds a *week*, because the timeframe of a week makes this goal a time-bound goal.

Now that we have discussed the *small wins strategy* and how to make *SMART Goals*, let's keep moving on. We have demonstrated the basics of establishing our goals and how to reward ourselves with things like a healthy, positive image, shopping spree, or simply a good report from the doctor from making our wise choices; now it's time to actually set up specific goals.

Step One

What do you want to accomplish? You have to know this before we can go any further. Do you want to lose weight, get a better looking body, become healthier, or simply feel better at any age? Once you specifically determine what you want to accomplish, we'll begin with our first step in setting up goals to proceed toward success.

Let's use some examples to help you through the process. Our first example will be to lose ten pounds. Now this is a very broad statement: "I want to lose ten pounds." OK—how do you do that? Let's start off with losing one to two pounds a week. This is a little more manageable than just the broad term, "lose ten pounds." So our first goal is to lose one to two pounds a week. How do we do this? Remember what we have already learned about *SMART Goals.* Stop right here and determine some specific goals and write them down. Yes—I want you to write them down in this book so they become real to you. You need to have a plan for success, and it will help you to commit if you write them down.

_____

_____

_____

_____

_____

_____

_____

Review

Let's step back for just a bit and take a look at what you wrote down above. Can you *measure* your *specific* goals? Come on—you know how to do this. Are you losing ten pounds or are you losing one to two pounds a week? Are your goals *aligned* with your overall goal? Are they *reachable and realistic?* Did you set a *timeframe?* Once you have made sure your goals are *SMART*, let's move on to the next step.

Step Two

Now it's time to break down our goals into *objectives.* Oh yeah, this is the other thing I studied in school. Basically, objectives are the little bitty methods you will use to achieve your overall goals. For example, your first goal of losing one to two pounds a week meets all of the criteria for a good, achievable goal. So *how* do you lose the one to two pounds a week? This is where objectives step in—keep asking yourself *how,* and you will understand how to write an objective.

For our example, we will begin by changing our nutrition plan slowly, eating breakfast or by substituting that fast food breakfast item for oatmeal topped with walnuts and blueberries (remember what we learned in the Nutrition Made Easy chapter). That's one of our objectives! Wasn't that easy? Another objective could be to eat five small meals instead of three large meals. We can break this down even further. Once we have our objectives of eating a healthy breakfast and five small meals a day, we could look specifically at our meal plan and break it down from there. These are *objectives* for our goal plan. Take just a moment and break down your first goal into some small objectives. Remember, objectives aren't goals; they are how you will accomplish your goal. Keep asking yourself *how.*

_____

_____

_____

_____

_____

Do you need my help? You can visit my Web site www.Fitness AnyAge.com for motivation and assistance with your goals and objectives. This is fun for me, and I want it to excite you, too. I know you will love it when you begin to see results.

Step Three

Now that you have established some very good measurable and attainable goals, and objectives as a pathway to reach them, you'll need to reward yourself. Remember our *small wins strategy?* It does work, ladies and gentlemen. We will assume you have passed your first week and lost one to two pounds of your overall goal; reward yourself. I don't mean by an ice cream sundae. How about treating yourself to a movie with a friend and sharing your victory? Or if you are feeling really good, try purchasing a new piece of clothing that fits a little better. It could even be something as simple as a new pair of sneakers so you can plow through the rest of your goals. Or if you're really ambitious, you could reward yourself by stepping up your goal plan and adding just one more repetition or one more round on your walk to your fitness plan; this is a *stretch goal*.

Whatever the reward, be kind to yourself. Show some appreciation, and motivate yourself to keep moving toward your goals. You have to love yourself or no one else can. Believe in you—take care of you. Today, tell yourself something great about you. Stop right now and write it down.

_____

_____

_____

_____

_____

_____

Ladies and gentlemen, my goal is to help you become healthier and fit at any age. In order to make this a specific and measurable goal, I have broken down my plan for accomplishing this goal through writing each chapter of this book. I hope you share the same appreciation that I have for goal setting. Ask any successful person, and they will all tell you they set goals for themselves. It doesn't matter if they are business goals or personal goals; goals are very effective at turning dreams into successes.

Closing Statement

This is truly the meat and potatoes (no pun intended) for our journey together—*goal setting*. I hope you have an understanding of how to set a goal using the steps for *SMART Goals*. Then always reward yourself using the *small wins strategy*. If you are really motivated, you can add in some *stretch goals* for additional motivation or to reach your goals faster.

First and foremost, learn to love yourself for who you are. None of us are the same; we are all different and come in all shapes and sizes. We will all have different goals and objectives for ourselves, and even have different goals at various stages in our lives. Just because I have a certain goal for myself does not mean you will share the same goal. Your goals are individual to you and your specific desires and needs. We are all special in our own way; don't forget to look for that, too. It's fine to *mirror* someone that you appreciate and do things this person does to achieve your own success. This is actually a good practice, as long as you don't lose *you* along the way. Now get with it, on your path to achieving your fitness goals today. Oops—I forgot to tell you something—you have to truly *believe in your goal*, too.

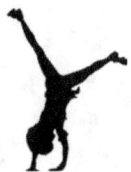

Competitions—Down and Dirty

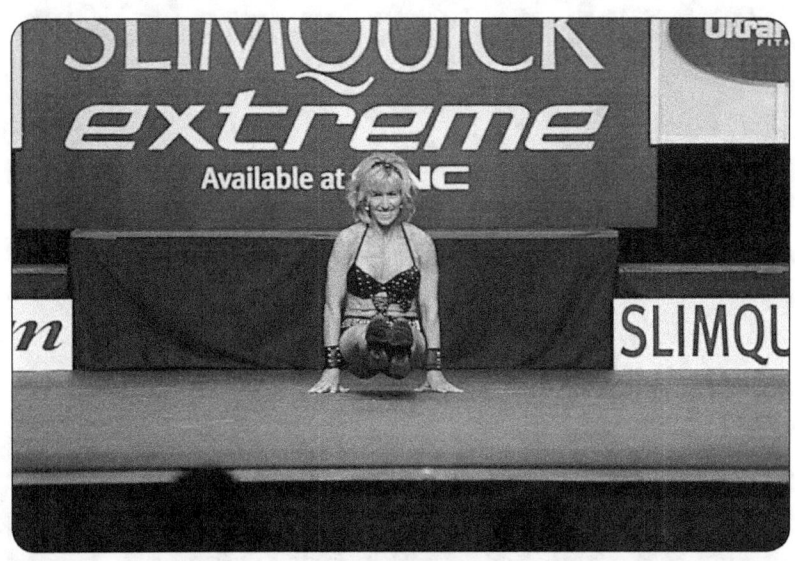

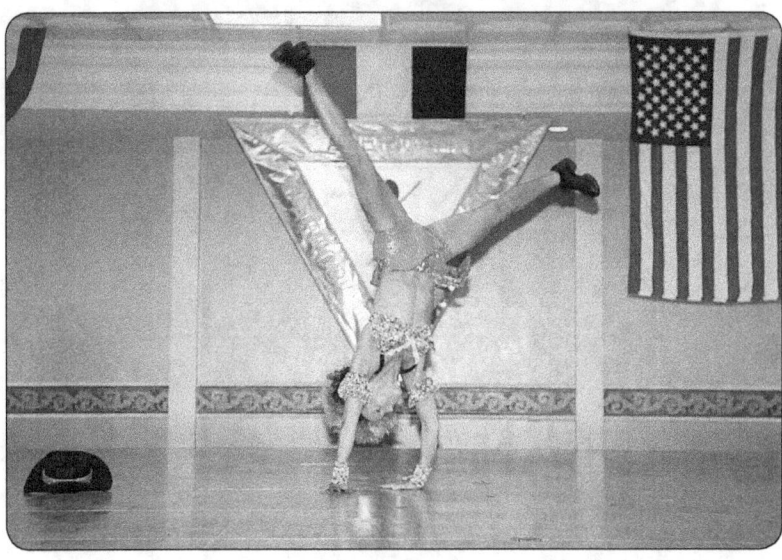

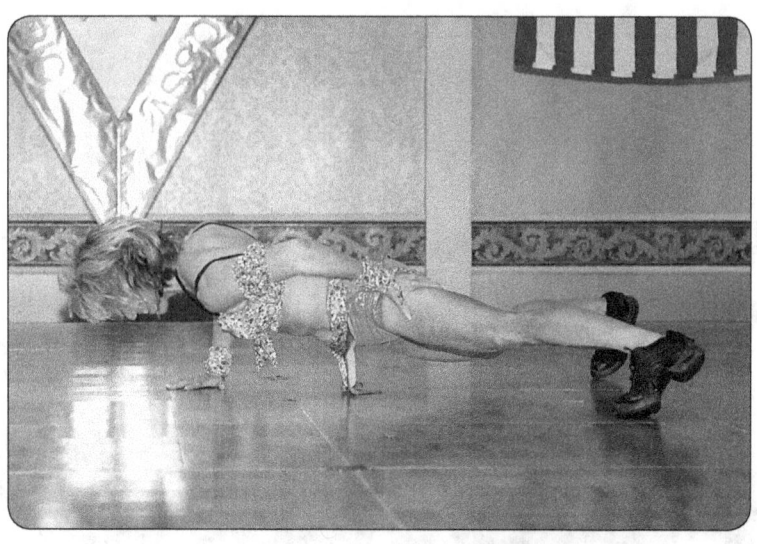

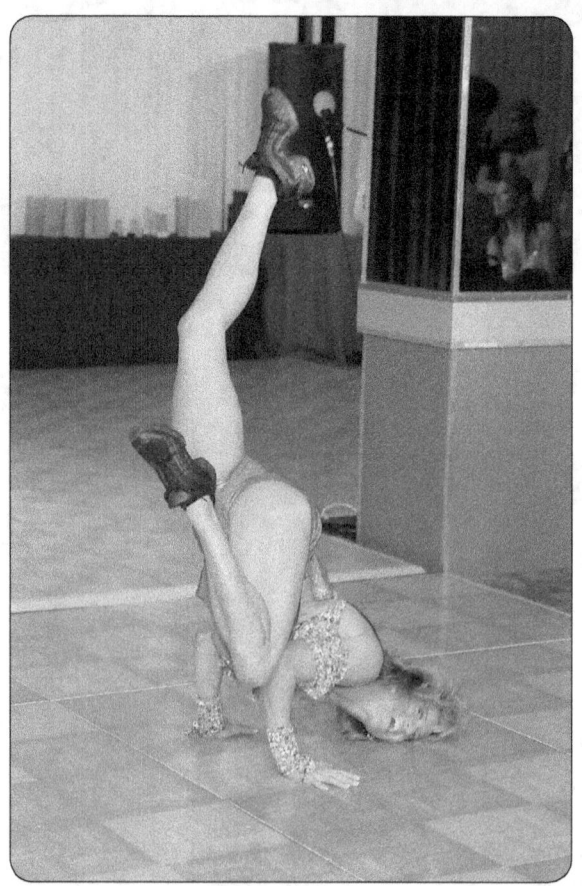

I have to admit; I couldn't wait to write this chapter, because competing in fitness shows is my absolute *passion*. In this chapter, I'm going to fill you in on the down and dirty of competition. You will learn what motivates people to compete, how they prepare, including training and nutrition (or diet down), plus the really nasty side of competition. So did that grab you enough to want to find out about the *nasty side?* Hold on…let's get started. It all begins with a *defining moment*.

Defining Moment

As you have learned by now, I've always been very active and try to eat a lot of the food groups considered to be nutritious. It all began back in September 2005 during a kickboxing class at a local Dallas gym. I always had so much fun doing kickboxing with this particular instructor because she utilized the famous techniques of the originator of Tae Bo. The instructor always looked very fit to me, but I began to notice something different about her appearance. Over a period of only a couple of weeks, her waistline appeared so much smaller and her muscle tone was also much more visible. Then one class day, she came in all tanned. I approached her after class, asking her how she got to look so good so quickly. She explained she was in training for a fitness competition the following week. I had never even heard of fitness competitions and was clueless as to what her training involved. When she returned from her competition, I was excited to hear how she placed. She had pictures of the competition and was showing everyone. She took first place at a local Dallas show, and her picture showed her holding a large bouquet of flowers, standing proudly in a tiny swimsuit and fake eyelashes. I told her she looked beautiful, and she did. Then I asked her who the young lady standing next to her in the swimsuit was, and my instructor said this woman had taken second place. I am sure at that very moment you could see stars in my eyes, because I looked at her and said very clearly, "Really?" She knew exactly what I was thinking and asked, "Sharon, are you thinking about competing?" I said, "Absolutely." That was it! I went home and announced to my husband, "Hey, honey, I am going to enter a fitness competition." He looked at me and said, "OK—what's that?" The rest is history. Do you see what I'm talking about now? That very moment with stars in my eyes was my *defining moment*.

We all have defining moments, but you have to **recognize it and grab on to it** while you are hot. If you don't, then it simply becomes a *fleeting moment* or a *wild idea* that never comes to fruition. Just think, if I had not recognized that I had a defining moment to compete and followed through with believing in myself, I wouldn't be telling you about it at this moment. By the way, the book you are holding in your hands was another critical defining moment.

Ever since I started competing, people ask me all the time what makes me do it and how I do what I do. They all want to know what to eat, how to exercise, and how to make commitments for healthier lifestyles. This is typically followed by, "You should really write all this down." Finally, one day in the middle of 2008, I was visiting with a gentleman from Austin, Texas, over the telephone about competition. He said, "You should write a book; you have a lot to say that people would be able to use." That was it! I had a *defining moment* again. I told him at that moment, "I am going to write a book," and I started that very week.

I think you get the gist. Learn to recognize your defining moment and follow through. Who knows…there are no limits as to what you, too, can accomplish. Let's get back to competition.

Training Camp

As I was following through with my dream to compete, my kickboxing instructor told me about a very cool fitness camp scheduled in Boston, Massachusetts, in January of 2006. So I booked a flight with her and off we went. I had an absolute blast. There were about two hundred girls in attendance, and I met some high-level top competitors in the industry, even though at the time I had no idea who they were. We learned how to eat, how to walk, how to talk, how to turn, how to stand, how to dance, and how to attempt to balance on one elbow. OK, the last one I still can't do. I borrowed a pair of what felt like eight-inch, clear, high heel shoes. You know the really high, clear shoes the strippers wear? OK, you know what I am talking about now. I couldn't even stand in those son of a guns, much less try and walk. It was ridiculous. EVERYONE was younger than I was, too. This was even more intimidating. Then I began to hear the girls' stories, and I very quickly felt different. There were young college girls, young mothers, older mothers (thirties and forties), a girl with a heart transplant, and girls with an eating disorder. I felt so lucky to be who I was.

I shared a room with two other girls, and there was lots of naked-ness, as you can imagine at a fitness camp. I became very comfortable with my body and the way I looked. Even approaching fifty, my boobs were just as good as or better than some. My butt was as good as or better than some. My confidence was also as good as or better than some. The thing I had in my favor in being the oldest was a strong belief in myself, and complete confidence that I could accomplish absolutely anything with dedication and training.

We had a ball in that room. One of the girls had competed several times and was telling us a story of how she was waxed the first time for the little bitty swimsuits, and we were all cracking up. To this day I have not had the courage to be waxed; I choose to shave during competitions. The waxing process sounds simply brutal.

The youngest girl in my room had a bottle of some sort of pills in her suitcase that she was taking as a drastic form of weight loss. Some of the other girls in attendance had physical builds that were more like guys than any girl I had ever seen. Hmm...do you think they were doing some sort of steroids? One had the deep voice to prove it. I was scared of her; she wore camouflage and combat boots. All the other girls knew her; I had no desire to.

The two most informative classes of training camp were the nutritional class and the walking class. The walking class involved putting on those ridiculous shoes and strutting. Some of the girls never took the plunge and had the courage to walk; I did. I strutted in my pink sweats, eight-inch high, clear shoes, and a sports bra top. Quite a sight—too funny. Then we had a follow up class in which we were sized up by the promoter to see where we stood in preparation for competition. I was shocked; I had the feeling she would think I was too old or not toned enough. She reviewed my body, told me I looked great, and said that a good nutritional plan would totally take care of my love handles. She said my color was pink (my absolute favorite color) for my swimsuit. I felt so special, like I had just won my first beauty contest. I took notes on everything for my file. One of the most disappointing things was I would have to give up real ice cream. I fully planned on substituting the light kind; at least, that is what I thought.

Nutrition Change – Diet Down

Understand one important thing right now. The chapter on nutrition is critical to your well-being and a healthier lifestyle. The diet down phase of competition is necessary and difficult for any competitor and should ONLY be used when competing. Luckily, I have always liked really healthy veggies, fish, and chicken. Unfortunately, I have always liked junk such as chocolate and candy, too. So I slowly began to make positive changes in my nutrition as I learned from the *nutritionist* at fitness camp. The important thing here is that I began to eat more frequent meals and cut back on portions and junk foods. I began to drop pounds; I started out around 128 pounds. It was a slow weight loss, which is the way you should do it. Next thing you knew, my tummy began to go down. I have always had a pooch—except right before competition and right after. I have learned that if you eat clean, you will not have a pooch. If you are interested on how I did it, please refer to the chapter on nutrition. It is a healthy approach to getting to your desired weight.

Everything went out the window as I got closer to my competition date, which was still about four months out. I stopped losing weight, and I didn't know what else to do based on what I thought I had learned. Then I heard about another local sports nutritionist in Dallas, so I went to her and paid a handsome two hundred dollars. What a joke—or so I thought! She printed out a bunch of stuff with supplement information that seemed very repetitive and even talked about steroids in the material. She placed me on a strict diet of so many ounces of this and that; what I thought was ridiculous at the time. I tried to stick to her diet, and I hated it. So I called the nutritionist in Boston and told her about my dilemma. She gave me some more pointers and changed up my program somewhat. It worked!

Remember, what I am about to tell you is NOT how you should eat under normal circumstances, even though it seems so healthy. No one can live like this very long, as it can get very boring.

The Secret Diet-Down Diet

I'm about to share my secret to looking like I do in competition. This diet lasts anywhere from three to four weeks, depending on how toned I look and if my pooch is still visible. With some people, this may take three to four months. I need to preface this with the fact that I make my lunch fresh every single morning to take to work, and I make extra food in the evening that I pack in small plastic containers to have as my snacks.

- 7:00 a.m. –Every single morning, I eat oatmeal covered in blueberries and/or and a few walnuts and three egg whites.
- 9:30 a.m. –Then around 9:30 a.m. (you need to eat every two to two and a half hours), I have either a piece of fish (or chicken) and broccoli. Yes, I said fish and broccoli! Cold! Trust me, after a while, this cold fish tastes pretty damn good.
- 1:00 p.m. –After my workout at noon, I have a large, green, leafy salad with spinach mix covered with baby carrots, small tomatoes, blueberries, one egg white, a pack of chunk light tuna, and a teaspoon of almond oil, with two, light, whole grain Wasa crackers.
- 1:15 p.m. – Two bite-sized pieces from a cut up protein bar. This is kind of like a piece of candy, but it is not quite as bad. I cut up a bar at the beginning of the week and place in a baggie in the refrigerator at work. I can't help it—I like candy. This makes my body think it is getting a piece of candy. At least I am getting a little more protein with a bite.

- 3:00 p.m. – Another piece of chicken breast or fish and a piece of broccoli or asparagus (this can be changed up). I have found yellow squash does not taste good cold, nor do my snacks taste good heated, so I eat them cold.
- 7:00 p.m. – By this time, I am starving! I have a piece of fish (salmon preferably), lots of green veggies and sometimes a piece of yellow squash, and a sweet potato almost every single night. This is fantastic for you. You can even add another small, green salad with dinner.
- 8:30 p.m. – As I get close to competition (one week out), I even add a small green salad or chicken and broccoli again before I settle down for the night. Works wonders.
- 8:45 p.m. – Sugar-free Jell-O with sugar-free whipped cream. Yes, this is my snack. This has to go away a week out from competition.
- Note – the closer I get to competition (a couple of days out), I will even eat white fish, asparagus, and a sweet potato for breakfast. I am so lean and basically starving from eating so frequently that this tastes fantastic. Seems odd that the more often I eat, the more I lose as long as it is the right types of foods.

Now you know my secret. Totally healthy—no drugs or supplements! Eating this way for up to eight weeks will ensure you will look fantastic. Your body can't help it; it will respond. It takes dedication like you wouldn't believe and lots of good cooking, which I don't do; my husband does that, and he looks great during my competitions, too. Even when I have to travel for business, he makes me mini-meals to take and packs them in ice containers to be checked at the airlines. I can eat the prepared meals for a couple of days after they are placed in a refrigerator. I even carry a small ice container in my car and eat small meals when I am driving. I carry a pre-made meal with me when I play golf while everyone else is having a beer and pizza. You have to make up your mind as to what you want and go for it. Needless to say, when I eat this way, I look exactly how I need to during the physique rounds at competition, even against girls twenty to thirty years my junior.

The Routine

Let's face it. I was going to be fifty years old for my first competition. I had never taken gymnastics, never been a cheerleader, never been on a drill team—nothing to prepare me for what I was about to embark upon. I hired a choreographer, who told me I had a long way to go. I hired a trainer, who basically told me I needed a year to prepare my body; she was also a competitor in muscle competitions. Very intimidating.

I went to the Cooper Aerobics Center in Dallas, Texas, every single Sunday for about a month to meet with my choreographer. I knew she was frustrated with me. I was very stiff (no flexibility) and couldn't remember any of her arm movements combined with the kicking and all sorts of stuff that appeared to be just like cheerleading from about thirty years ago. I even videotaped her and would watch while trying the moves in my living room daily with my glasses perched on my nose. I just couldn't get it to save my life. Finally, she hit me with what seemed like a shotgun to the face. She said, "I just can't work with you." I WAS DEVASTATED! I told her I completely understood and went home. In tears, I told my husband. But even hearing that, I didn't give up. The choreographer mentioned a girl she knew by the name of Micaela Brigida. I was so excited, because I already knew Micaela from the health club.

I approached Micaela the following week after class with my dream for competing, and she also devastated me when she informed me she had retired from teaching. She asked me if I could do a one-arm pushup or a pike. Of course, I couldn't do either; I didn't even know what a pike was. She said, "I never even consider working with someone until they can do a one-arm pushup." Then she did something miraculous; she got down on all fours in the dressing room of the club and placed a trash container underneath one arm, showing me how to practice to be able to do a one-arm pushup. I asked her to please reconsider, as she was my only hope. She saw the desire in my eyes and said she would come out of retirement just one more time for me. She said it was because of my age and desire that "Fitness Is for Any Age." She was the first choreographer to actually believe in me.

We signed a contract and began meeting the following week. Micaela played my music ("Boots Are Made for Walking" and "She's Got Legs") and showed me a couple of very sexy moves with a straw hat, and a simple turn-around with a foot movement completed by a hip drop. I did it. She informed me that I had my first element. I literally had tears in my eyes when I said proudly, "I have my first element." The rest is history. I worked so hard learning, and I practiced EVERY SINGLE DAY in my living room, watching my videotape of what Micaela taught me just to make her proud when we would meet. Even though I wore kneepads, I had bruises on my knees, hips, and arms. I dropped on my head and tailbone. But I made progress, and I had a routine. I had to stretch, stretch, and then stretch again every single day.

The routine was so cute, too—my favorite so far. People called the routine "Boots." Then Micaela made me perform the routine in front of her cardio class at Lifetime Fitness in Plano. I was terrified! No spray tan and white as a ghost in my little outfit with leggings that made me look like Peter Pan. I performed the routine, and then she made me talk. The class started asking me questions as I stood there with a microphone; I was so scared and vulnerable. They saw my passion and became a part of it, and it flowed after that. I was so hooked. I love Micaela to this day for what she did for me and for her belief in me. I knew I could do it, and she knew I could, too. We continued to practice every single week, and she designed a costume for me and colors for a swimsuit. Then she told me about an opportunity to get in front of the judges, which she said would be a good thing for me to do before the big event.

I called the director of the judges for the event, and he talked me into going to perform my routine and speak. I had my husband and son go with me to videotape it. I look back at that tape now, and I was so awful. It seems so long ago, and yet it is so precious, the very accomplishment of following through on such an adventure. There were only two competitors, and of course I came in second. I wore a huge, beautiful, Academy Awards-type dress and had my hair up with sparkly earrings on. I felt so special, and my husband was so proud.

The director called me that night saying I was now *qualified* to compete in Ms. Fitness USA, and there was still time to book flights. I told my husband that I was going to jump at the opportunity. So this meant I had to practice very hard with Micaela on the routine before I went to compete. I was probably as good as I was going to be at this point, being so new.

Weight Training

Another critical part of training for a fitness competition is weight training. Some competitors do not train with weights; some simply utilize plyometrics as their form of training and that's OK, too. I needed weight training to get my body toned where it needed to be in order to be able to compete well in the physique round. The more I dieted down and trained with weights, the better I looked each day. I developed a six-pack for the first time in my whole life, and people began to notice. No one believed me, of course, when they asked why I was losing weight and looking so good. People are very skeptical when you tell them you are training for a fitness competition at fifty. My trainer was even skeptical at first, as she was ten years younger than I was. All of that simply fueled me to prove that I can. I trained with my trainer once a week very hard for an hour and then utilized what she taught me and incorporated it into my own routine throughout the week. So I was performing in a boot camp-type class on Monday, kickboxing on Tuesday, meeting with my trainer on Wednesday, yoga and stretching on Thursday, and weight training again on Friday. I would then meet with my choreographer on the weekends. I forgot to mention that I practiced my routine every single night right after work. I was exhausted and bruised but determined at fifty. And I had never looked so good in all my life!

As I got closer to competition, I had to train with the weights twice a week for a few weeks to get that extra pump I needed for my muscles. My body began to respond. Plus, my trainer began to believe in me, knowing full well I was going to do it. Let me tell you, it hurts! Once you start doing physical stuff to your body like I was doing at fifty, it really hurts. You have heard the old song, "Hurts So Good"? That is how I felt. It was all worth it. My body became so toned and lean and strong. I finally mastered the one-arm pushup beautifully with no problem. I could even hold the pushup in the down position—awesome for my age. I still cannot believe I did that. The company I worked for even put it on their Web site. I became known in the Dallas brokerage community as the senior property manager who could do a one-arm pushup. My son would challenge all of his friends to a one-arm pushup, saying, "My mom can do one and you can't."

Spray Tanning

Another very important step in competing is spray tanning. I absolutely do not recommend baking in the sun or in the tanning booth. Please stay away from these two drastic steps as a last resort to preparing for a fitness competition. I tried the sponge-on products, and they were just awful! They stain not only your skin but will spot the floor, clothing, sheets, heels, elbows, and whatever else gets in their way. I was first introduced to the sponge-on type at Ms. Fitness USA. I e-mailed one of the top well-known competitors and told her I was brand new and didn't know anybody to help me. She was a doll and agreed to help. She told me when I arrived in Vegas to call her after I had completely showed and scrubbed my skin—with no lotion. I remember scrubbing myself completely, wrapping my towel around me, my hair up with no makeup, answering the door. She walked in; I shook her hand and introduced myself. I dropped my towel and was butt naked a minute later, and she was sponging this nasty stuff all over my whole body. I mean spread-eagled so the dark tanner got into every single nook and cranny that you can possibly imagine. You have to do this, or you will not look good on stage. Then you cannot shower until the next evening or it will all come off and you have to do it again. After a competition, I would let the water run over my body and pat dry; the stuff comes off easily on the towels and sheets, so you have to carry your own to a competition so you don't ruin the hotel's linens. I learned to wash my hair in the sink, too.

Then I discovered the beauty of getting a competition spray tan. You have a whole bunch of naked girls in a room with hair in towels getting sprayed down and standing bent-over while another girl blows the body dry with a hair dryer. This also makes a horrible mess in the girl's room. As I mentioned before, competition is a lot of nakedness—you just get used to it. The person that sprays you will see every SINGLE place on your body that no one else sees, except maybe your gynecologist! After you dry, you have to sleep in very loose fitting pajamas, especially around the waist. If you don't, you will do exactly what I did and place your hands on your stomach and wake up with finger prints on your belly and have to be repainted. For one competition, I looked like I was a black woman instead of a white woman—no kidding. On stage, it was beautiful.

The spray tanning is a very expensive process but the absolute way to go. For my short and quick shows, I carry a can of competition spray tan in my bag, wrapped in a plastic bag in case it explodes. My husband has to spray me down before I leave the day before for a really good base, and then I attempt to spray myself after I get in town. This is challenging if you don't have anyone that can help out. Trust me—no funny business either when you have been sprayed. It does come off, ladies and gentlemen. That kind of stuff can wait until after competition and you have showered, mainly because you stink! Not only does the spray stink, but you cannot wash your important parts or underarms. Your special parts stink! I carry a box of baby wipes so I can at least wash the very important parts—not the underarms, or you will have huge white marks underneath your arms when you raise them. And to use the bathroom—why do you even ask me! Ladies, you'll have to basically straddle the toilet to pee in an effort to keep the tanner from being accidentally splashed and coming off of your inner thighs. Plus the tanner gets on the toilet seat, too. Yuck!

Swimsuit, Dress, and Jewelry

Depending upon the federation and the competition you are entering, all of these things become critical. You must know each federation's rules and regulations relating to what you can and cannot wear. Also, you need to learn what the judges look for. I have competed in many different competitions underneath different federations, and they are all looking for something different. Plus, it is so political. Some of them know who the winner is before the competition even begins, depending upon the sponsor of the show—or who sleeps with whom, unfortunately.

The swimsuit is different for each competition; how much cheek and boob you can show. The same goes for the routine outfit. The Ms. Fitness USA competition will not allow much cheek or boob, whereas most of the other federations want as much as you can put out there. This is where I got into trouble with the back of the swimsuit in trying to keep my estrogen patch covered up on my butt cheek. Some of the girls use a bikini bite or tape to keep things in place.

A lot of the federations are now requiring an evening gown speaking round, which is wonderful. This round is critical to seeing how well poised the model is and how well she speaks in front of an audience. Makeup, hair, nails, and jewelry become critical in this type of competition. The judges will even comment if they like your hair or if they like a certain piece of jewelry. I was called down one time from a judge who said I clicked my nails, when all I was doing was counting the points in my speech so I could remember. Everything is scrutinized; competing is not for the weak-natured. One of the most important things they look for is how relaxed you are, not necessarily what you are saying. They want sincerity more than a prepared speech.

The Walk and Posing

Thankfully, I learned how to walk and turn in competition from a pro. Then I purchased a DVD and practiced in my living room in my competition heels again and again. The walk becomes critical, as well as how to perform a turn. This depends upon the federation, too, as to how much priss you can add and get away with. The Fitness America Pageant wants as much priss and confidence as possible in their walk and turn. Ms. Fitness USA wants a calmer, more reserved clock turn. You have to understand what the judges are looking for before you go to any competition; read anything you can get your hands on before entering.

I learned a smile goes a long way in any competition. Some of the federations do not put much emphasis on this, but I have always done it anyway. The judges will remember when you flash your pearly whites at them. Don't stare them down, either. Glance over and acknowledge the judges, and then turn back away and face forward with your line. The judges consider a stare intimidating. They are judging your body. I use whitening strips before any competition to give my teeth an extra edge.

With experience and practice in front of a mirror, you will learn which of your poses looks the best and will score the highest for pictures. You will develop poses that will be your own *winning poses*. I have noticed in my family holiday pictures that my body automatically will go into a competition pose; it comes naturally now. The walk and turn is another opportunity to turn around and flash a winning smile and pose. You never know; a judge may score you a little higher for the turn and pose. Cock the heel just a bit to show the calf muscle; not too high, though. And then relax, or the judges will call you down for posing in the line. They like you to be relaxed.

Mental Games

I have won a lot of competitions (both first and second place); I have even won mentally when I came in last place. It is all in how you feel about it. I know I am an automatic winner the minute I set foot on that stage. I know what it takes to walk out on to stage and either perform or speak. Before I go up to do either, I picture myself actually doing the performing. I also picture myself getting the first-place trophy. I can't tell you how many times it felt surreal that I had actually lived through the process even before it happened, because I saw it in my mind. I had accepted the trophy in my mind many times before I actually won. It is really weird, but it works.

Closing Remarks on Competitions

Competition is about believing in yourself and who you are and what you can accomplish. It is about passion and commitment. It is about not allowing anyone to set your limitations for you. It is about having faith in your abilities and trusting your instincts and your defining moments enough to take the plunge and go for it. After all, what do you have to lose? Think about it. I had a little girl about eight years old come up to me and ask for my autograph after that first big competition in Vegas, when I walked offstage in my big black Academy Award-like dress. No kidding—me! Her mother then excitedly told me I had inspired them. If I could do it, then maybe they could, too. Times like that I will never forget. I felt like a movie star, and I felt like a winner. If you look at the stats for that particular competition, I was at the bottom. I was also the oldest. Didn't matter to me; I have won many first place trophies since that night, but I'll also never forget that first night and my first competition. I was a winner and still am. So are you, no matter what your pursuit is in life—as long as you believe and attempt to do it. In my book, that makes you a winner.

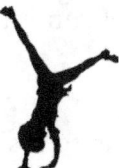

Challenges and Focus

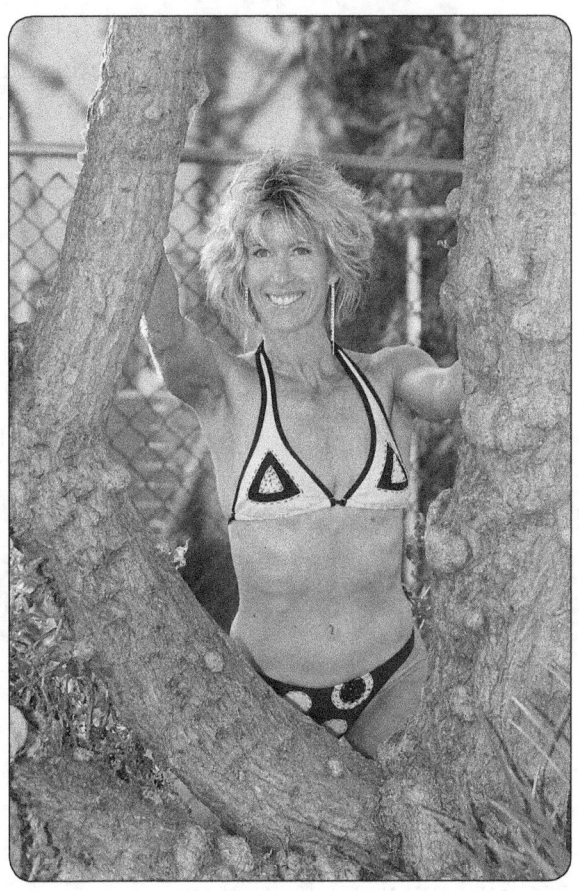

Life is going to present challenges for each of us every single day, so this is not a sad violin song from me. That is not the purpose of us spending this valuable time together. Let's review our purpose, so we can then discuss challenges that all of us face at one point or another in each of our lives. The purpose of this book is to offer a basic plan for a healthier lifestyle and to prove to you that YOU CAN DO IT—you just have to believe and have a commitment to your goal, whatever that goal might be.

I wanted to begin this chapter with an incredible story of dedication, passion, and commitment to a single focus—to succeed. This story shows that **Fitness Is for Any Age** and **Age Is Simply a State of Mind**. It first hit the media in 2008 on *Good Morning America* and other broadcasts, including local news stations. The story was appropriately delivered in the March 2009 issue of *Runner's World Magazine* and featured Paul Gionfriddo. This incredible gentleman ran his first 5-K race at sixty and continued running marathons across the U.S. until he finished his one hundredth marathon. Then, in honor of his eight-sixth birthday, he ran a 50-K. He did cross that finish line.

Another wonderful story was featured in the *Dallas Morning News* online (www.DallasNews.com) on March 12, 2009, by columnist Steve Blow. Ms. Fan Benno-Caris was over the news, talking about her run for the Addison City Council at ninety-one years of age. That's right! She is ninety-one years young. Ms. Benno-Caris started *race walking* when she was seventy and fell in love with it since it resembled the rumba. She also took dance lessons and loved them. Ms. Benno-Caris stated on a local television news station that she felt twenty-one years young. She said she lived through the Depression and knew how to save money, and therefore felt she could do a good job serving on the City Council.

The reason I wanted to highlight these two stories is to illustrate that **Fitness Is for Any Age** and **Age Is Simply a State of Mind**. While most of us, including me, may see what these two individuals have accomplished as an impossible challenge, these two incredible people see their *challenge* as their passion. Remember, they never let anyone else set their limitations for them.

I want to focus on how we view the challenges we face throughout our lives and help to put them into perspective. You know the old saying "one man's trash is another man's treasure"? Well, this is sort of the same philosophy. Our "impossible challenge" may be viewed by someone else as an "absolute passion." That is exactly how I view being a fitness competitor over the age of fifty! It is my absolute passion, and I do not even acknowledge roadblocks; at least, I won't give them the time of day—I just go around them. I can't repeat enough that **Fitness Is for Any Age** and **Age Is Simply a State of Mind.**

Physical Challenges

Let me share with you a truly amazing story that I personally witnessed at a fitness show held in Plano, Texas, in September 2006. There was a young fitness competitor in her twenties who didn't have any **arms**! Yes, you heard me right; she didn't have any arms, and she was competing against girls with arms. It was the most amazing thing I have ever witnessed. This girl didn't allow her personal challenge to interfere with her absolute passion—her love for fitness. She was able to do things that were unimaginable, including flips and the splits. She took second place in the competition, and she inspired me to compete in this same competition the following year.

I know some of you have physical challenges that may inhibit your pursuit of a healthier lifestyle, but please don't let that stop you from trying. You probably feel there is no hope and you can't possibly get out of your house and do some of these things. How do you know until you try? I am not suggesting that you run out and enter a fitness competition; I am suggesting that you get up and try to walk or do something that will help you feel better about yourself. Exercise is an amazing thing, both physically and mentally. If your personal challenge doesn't allow you to get up and walk, try something within your range of possibilities that will allow you to challenge the impossible.

There is a second story that I want to share about another young fitness competitor who I personally watched in Boston. She had a heart transplant shortly before the competition. She had slowly recovered and continued the pursuit of her passion—to compete. I have kept up with her story over the last several years, and she is still competing and doing very well. Then there is my friend and fellow competitor out of Alaska who had breast cancer a few years ago and survived. Her only thought was, "How do I get back into competitions?" and she was upset she couldn't do the one-arm pushup. That's inspirational!

The reason I am sharing these stories with you is so we can begin to focus more on what we can do instead of what we can't do. Don't you think that is a much more productive choice?

Injuries and Surgeries

Most of us who pursue an exercise program, fitness program, or sport will encounter injuries and/or surgeries. This is so challenging; trying to recover and then the mental game of not being at your best and having to take it easy. It drives me crazy. One year before I made the decision to compete in my first fitness competition, I had a complete hysterectomy! That's right. I had eight golf ball-sized tumors and some other female issues that were swelling my abdomen to a size of what appeared to be a first trimester pregnancy. Look at some of my competition pictures, and you wouldn't think that—right? Well, I was so depressed and felt there was no hope of ever getting back to normal; I was also afraid of being cut. The doctor was able to perform a bikini cut hysterectomy, so there was very little scarring and it isn't even visible in a show bikini. This was a blessing considering my passion was fitness. I was under strict orders from the doctor to not move whatsoever from my living room for six weeks and not even consider touching a weight. The day after my doctor released me at six weeks, I was back at the gym. I was back in my triathlete-type training within two weeks. Then I began training for my first fitness competition held one year later.

Last year during a practice session, I turned a cartwheel that didn't feel quite right. My next move was to turn around and go into a handstand, and I almost walked straight over in my bend; so I fell over sideways. I was a bit dizzy and knew something wasn't quite right. My right shoulder hurt a bit later that day, but I didn't think too much about it. I was in the midst of training for a competition only three weeks out. I headed off to the competition, but my shoulder gradually got worse. So what did I do? I headed off to a second competition the following month, and it again got worse. Within two months, I began physical therapy for what doctors thought was a "frozen shoulder." Four months later with it not getting better, the doctor ordered an MRI and confirmed a torn rotator cuff with hardened capsule. Wow! I had been competing with these two challenges, knowing something wasn't quite right but not allowing it to interfere with my passion and love of fitness. I don't recommend this; I wasn't aware I had a torn rotator cuff. I am now in recovery.

I remember how depressed I was when the doctor showed me the MRI slide, thinking I wouldn't be able to compete again. Let's face it; I was fifty-two at the time, approaching fifty-three years young. I didn't have a lot of time left for surgery and then recovery. Most fitness competitors quit the sport in their mid-forties—much less fifty! Then the doctor told me he wouldn't limit my activities only if I understood that I couldn't "fall" while performing; he said surgery could come later. So the goal was to modify the routine so it didn't include moves where I could possibly fall and tear the shoulder out— all because of my passion for fitness. I went to the gym right after my doctor's appointment to lift weights again, and mentally it was such a boost that I can't explain.

Mental Games

Let's talk about that last statement—mental games. Nothing had changed with my arm from the time I walked into the doctor's office until an hour later when I left. It was a mental game when the doctor told me I could compete again and he wouldn't limit me. I told him that day, "Doctor, I want to be on that stage in September." He said there was no reason I wouldn't be. I felt invincible again like I could do it, and I did. This is what I am trying to get across to you. Believe in yourself and set out to accomplish whatever your goal might be. Tell yourself you can do it, and then believe it. Talk to a trusted friend who is positive and ask them to encourage you; avoid negativity.

Sure, it hurts like hell! My right arm wakes me up during the night, and now my left arm is hurting in the same places from over-compensating, most likely. I don't complain; I just keep moving. I never forget the girl without any arms competing in a fitness competition, and I THANK GOD I even have arms. This is what it is all about—praise God for the things you do have no matter what those things are. It could be a lot worse. I immediately began to train to compete for the fourth year and my eleventh fitness competition! I am mastering the left one-arm pushup—not only one pushup but three on the same side. This shows what passion and commitment and a burning desire to succeed can do. I am proof that fitness can come at any age, and you can be fabulous over fifty!

Focus and Commitment

I firmly believe you can do anything you set your mind to as long as you believe in yourself. You have to have pride, passion, and commitment to surround your dreams and goals. Focus on whatever it is that you want to do—follow the steps in this book to establish your goals and objectives for success—then do it! This is the commitment part—you have to actually do it (stop just talking about it).

Oh, there is something very important that I need to remind you at this point in our journey together. **Don't allow anyone to set your limitations for you!** I can't say that statement loudly enough. You know how negative people can be; they can even be jealous and will cut you down. If you are overweight and begin to lose weight, you know that people will actually tell you looked better overweight. Or they will start saying bad things about you or even encourage you to eat bad food again. Some will try to sabotage your journey. That is their problem; don't let it stop you from bettering yourself. Ignore them and move forward.

This is the focus portion—moving forward. Put on those blinders and don't let anyone stop you from achieving your dreams, whatever they might be. Don't kid me; you have dreams. I know you do, and you do, too. Even if you have become depressed and think you'll never get back in those jeans, or walk down the street, or enter a health club and feel comfortable without everyone staring at you (or so you think), you can do it! No matter what your personal challenge is, make a decision right now to change the way you are thinking and focus on how to overcome your challenge and make it a passion instead.

I want you to stop right now and write down what you feel your *greatest challenge* is and commit to at least try to overcome this challenge. This is the first step—to recognize it.

_____

_____

_____

_____

Now that we have established your greatest challenge and you have committed to try to overcome it, go back and put a date by it. In a week, I want you to come back to this page and review what you have committed to and make sure you have taken the first step to overcome. Remember all the steps in the book; this will help you with your commitment and plan of action.

Failure? Not!

There will come times when you think you have not made any progress and that you have *failed*. NOT! *Fail* is a four-letter word that we will never say again. If you don't try, then you will never know—right? That would be the greatest loss—to not try and then not know. I like to look at it as a test. I have always said that God provides us with little bitty tests each day of our lives to help prepare us for the big exam. So they aren't failures; they are simply little tests, and then we try again for the next test. Once we take all the tests and then take the exam, it starts over again, sort of like in school. So get with it and start preparing for your first test. Do your homework and make some commitments, set your goals and objectives for success, and never allow anyone to set your limitations for you. The sky is the limit! Let's see what others have to say about their goals and successes in the next chapter.

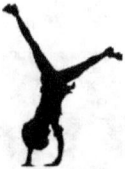

Testimonials

This chapter is meant to move and inspire you by sharing stories from others who believe that Fitness Is for Any Age and Age Is Simply a State of Mind. You can be Fifty, Fit, and Fabulous! I would like to start with a very dear friend of mine who has always believed in me and in my pursuit of fitness and writing.

Bob Kinsey, Lancaster, Texas

Wow! Sharon, talk about inspirational. You are a living testimonial to goal accomplishment. I noticed and understand why you did not dwell on your successful business career in your book. If your readers understood your accomplishments in that field while pursuing your avocation of fitness, they would really be amazed. I say keep up the good work. How does one achieve the dedication necessary to accomplish such high standards? Finding that desire is key. People tend to make excuses why they don't find success. I am a firm believer that darn near anything can be accomplished if we really "want" it badly enough. To know you and to be a small part of your journey has been my good fortune. I think your title is an excellent choice, and we both know that you are a great example of what can be achieved if an individual follows a program that fits his or her lifestyle. Since I am retired, I have implemented your program from the book. My activity level is still strong and I still fly my airplane, travel, work in the yard, and play with the grandsons every chance I get. I do support your efforts and am sure you will succeed.

Avis Petty, Mesquite, Texas, 45 years young

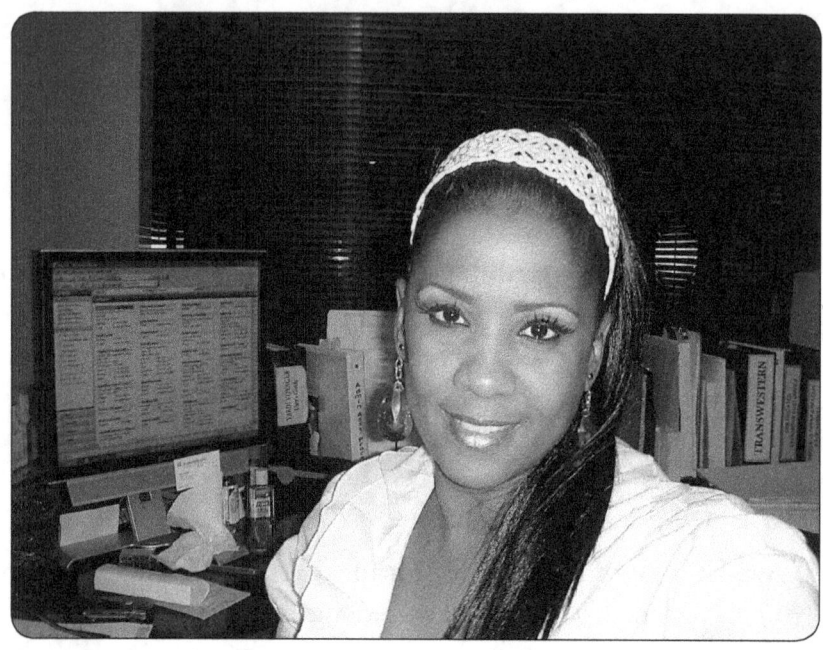

Over the years, my life had become very stressful. Being married to a pastor who has two churches in two states and is a motivational speaker, and being a mother and working a full-time job had overwhelmed me to where I lost control of my life and health. It seemed like it just happened suddenly. My eating habits had been reduced to eating out or eating late. However, with this pattern, I was losing control and feeling depressed because my weight was off the charts. I was always tired and complaining about everything. In 2005, I met Sharon Simmons and became her assistant. I must say, the first day we met, there was a chemistry that was electrifying and authentic.

During that time I was forty pounds overweight—and yes, it is easy to do that when you are not disciplined. However, after coming in contact with Sharon as my boss and confidant, I had no other choice but to make some changes. Seeing her smiling and having so much energy every day, I realized that I had the smile but not the energy. I watched her daily, as she was committed to working out and eating healthy. At that time, I couldn't understand why she would eat a small salad with a little oil instead of my idea of a perfect lunch, which was a hamburger and fries. Nevertheless, the results were very noticeable.

One day, I approached Sharon after she returned from her daily workout to find out what her method was to maintaining her weight. She gave me an eating plan and a workout program that would fit into my busy schedule. I followed her plan, and it did work. This gave me so much joy that I shared her plan with my husband and my seventy-one-year-old mother-in-law, and they saw results, too. I lost over forty pounds and I am able to manage my daily tasks effectively.

I feel good about the results that have taken place in my life due to my commitment and discipline to be fit. I relate this to 1 Corinthians 6:19–20, which reads, *"Our bodies are the temple of the Holy Spirit who is in us, and we don't belong to ourselves, but we have been bought with a price and we must use our bodies for the glory of God."* I thank God for allowing my path to cross with Sharon's, because it was her commitment and endurance that gave me the desire to take control of my life. Thank you, Sharon, and may God continue to bless you as you bless others.

Linda Mitchell, Ohio, 46 years young

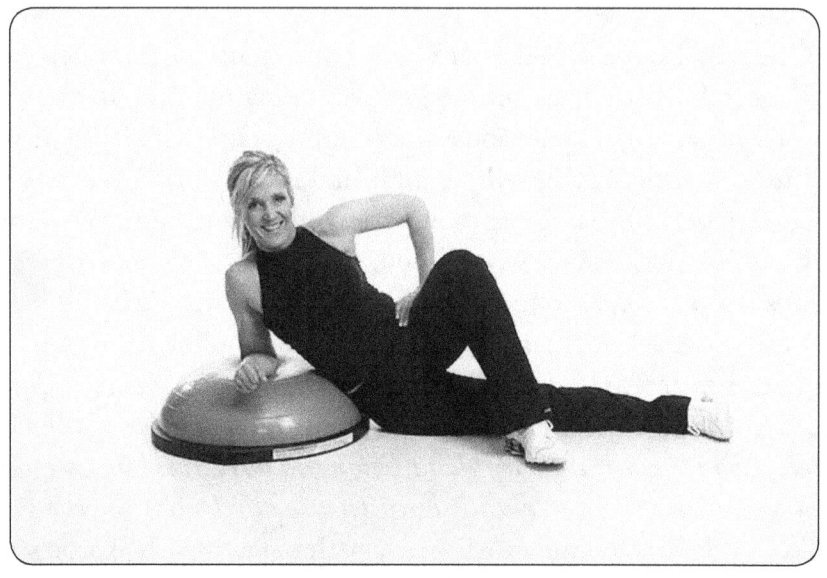

Fitness is not only a lifestyle; it is also a career, a way of life, and very much my passion. As a mother of three children ages twenty-six, twenty-four, and eleven, I began competing at the age of thirty-eight and achieved the crowns of Ms. Fitness Indiana 2008, Ms. Fitness Kentucky 2008, Ms. Fitness Great Lakes 2002 & 2004, and Ms. Fitness Legacy Masters Champion. I am a Fit Mom Who Loves Fitness. I met Sharon Simmons while competing at Ms. Fitness USA competition, and we have continued our friendship, as we share the same fitness goals. I am a prime example that with hard work, determination, perseverance, and especially spirit, anyone can overcome and work through anything to get to where they want to be!

Photo is courtesy of Linda's daughter, Tiffany D. Krumpack.

Lisa Buchanan, Coppell, Texas, 48 years young

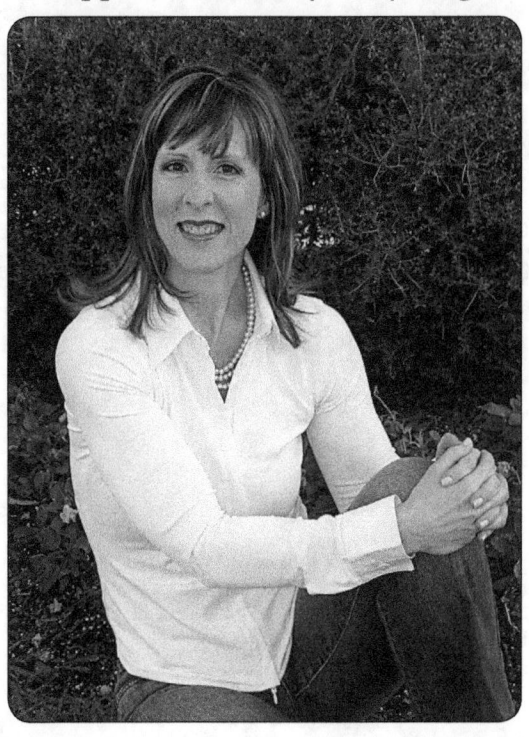

How my path led to caring deeply for the physical and mental health of others came from my own issues in those areas. I grew up in a Southern town with Southern foods. When you add to those family recipe genes that tend to be super-sized with gravy as a side, the result was a 145-pound frame with a wardrobe of size fourteens and sixteens. When I was nineteen, I decided that I was going to get into shape. That was a different way of thinking that involved a much more active mode of living compared to our sedentary school choir and Bible club in Chattanooga, Tennessee.

Back in the seventies, by walking, cutting out breads and desserts, and trying to follow the new aerobic trend, I dropped to 120 pounds and a size six. It was common sense, and I knew that it needed to become a way of life. Those changes fascinated me. Right before my eyes, I gradually changed—all because I made some simple choices and stayed consistent.

These days at the age of forty-eight, I weigh 143 pounds and I'm still a size six. There must be something to muscle being more dense than fat. This proves that weight is not the issue—it is the content!

In August of 2006, my husband and I made the decision to open *Fit by Design*, my own personal training and massage studio. This is where I met Sharon Simmons and witnessed her journey training and competing in fitness competitions. Remembering that it is God's business in the first place keeps me grounded and opens up many opportunities for changing lives.

Howard McKay (43 years young), RN, MSN, FNP-C, CPNP-AC
Nurse Practitioner, Double Board Certified
Honored–Great 100 Nurses, Dallas/Ft. Worth Metroplex 2009

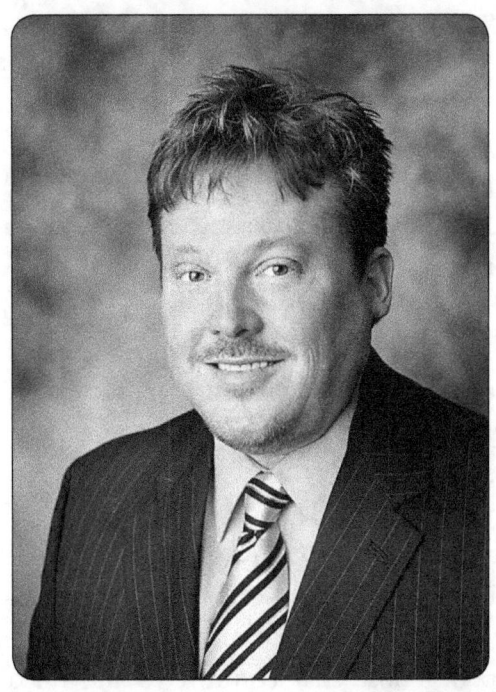

I have the great pleasure in my career to wear several different hats. Currently, I work as an acute care pediatric nurse practitioner at a local children's hospital, serve as an assistant clinical professor in a graduate school nurse practitioner program, and work with a very distinguished group of plastic surgeons in their skincare and laser center. So Fitness at Any Age is truly something very close to me, as I work with the entire spectrum of ages.

Being fit means so many different things. Many of us become fit physically, as we challenge our "machine" to run at high performance. Some of us challenge our minds to function at higher levels, and some of us search for a spiritual state of utopia.

As we must keep our inside healthy and our outside tone, we must also consider and keep our skin, hair, nails, grooming, wardrobe, cleanliness and outward demeanor polished at all times.

A diet rich in fruits, vegetables, lean protein and complex car-bohydrates is essential. Drinking plenty of water is also critical for hydration of the body. Fish oil, particularly those high in Omega 3 fatty oils, are essential to helping maintain elasticity of the skin and supporting good hair and nail growth. Skincare, as we age, is an evolving process. We know that if you do one thing, starting as an infant, is sunscreen, sunscreen, sunscreen!

For those that wish to look as young as they feel, dermal fillers and other products can be used to soften lines, provide a lift to the brow and prevent additional lines from forming on parts of the face. Laser procedures are options for more aggressive and longer-lasting correction. And, for those needing aggressive correction, traditional plastic surgical options are always available. However, if you are truly "fit", from the inside out, surgery can often be delayed until much later if not avoided completely.

I know truly that to be fit at any age is a very achievable state. I know this because I see it in my practice every day. Sharon Sim-mons is a glowing example of this! She is "Triple F – Fifty, Fit and Fabulous." One must have the commitment and mindset, however, to make it happen. Those that commit to and make total fitness a reality for themselves will and do live long and happy lives and shine like stars!

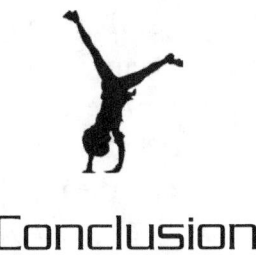

Conclusion

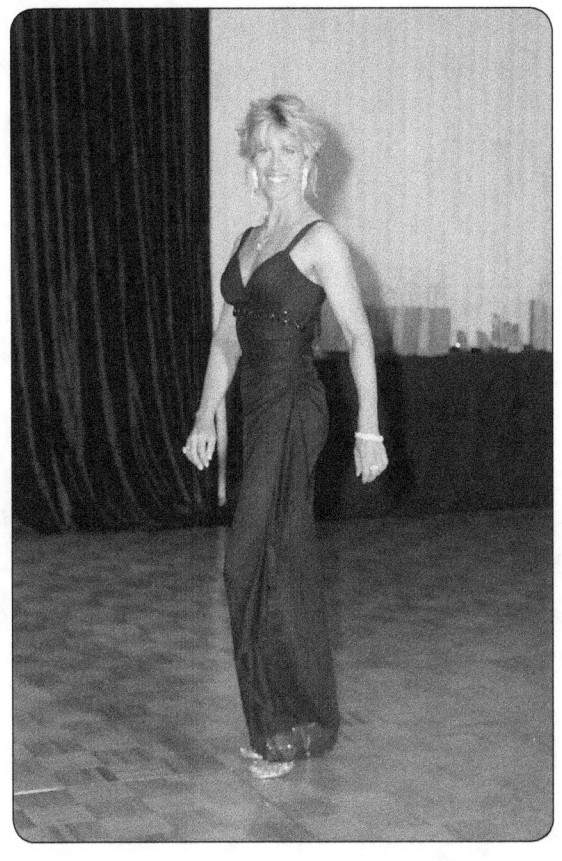

Hopefully, your journey through *Triple F: Fifty, Fit, and Fabulous* has been inspiring and has provided you with the necessary tools to live a healthier lifestyle. By now, you should have a basic plan for the two key ingredients needed to accomplish your fitness goals: nutrition and exercise. Remember, you have to have pride, passion, and commitment to a better you, and a burning desire to succeed at your goals. We have walked through the steps for goal setting and discussed some of the challenges that we may be faced with, along with suggestions to overcome them. Never allow anyone to set your limitations; only you can determine that. How do you know you can't succeed unless you try, and then try again? When others ask, "Why," respond, "Why not?" and then go for it! What do you have to lose? Learn to recognize your *defining moment* and make it a reality. Remember, you always have a friend who will listen and encourage you at www.FitnessAnyAge.com. Good luck with your new adventure, and may God bless you.

Sharon Simmons
Triple F: Fifty, Fit, and Fabulous!

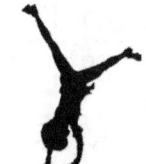

Thanks To:

Thanks to my loving husband, Scott Simmons, who has provided me with continued encouragement and emotional support during my educational pursuits, fitness goals and competitions, and now my writing career. Thank you for taking care of me. I love you.

Thanks to my son and my daughter for teaching me and reminding me about what being young at heart is all about. Also, for allowing me to be a kid with you as we struggled during each of your childhoods to make ends meet while making it fun. Thank you both for allowing me the privilege of being your mom and forgiving me when I didn't do that job perfectly. Thanks to my daughter for bringing two beautiful grandchildren into our family unit and for inspiring the title of my first book. Thank you to my son for always cheering the loudest when his mom was standing on the fitness competition stage.

Extended thanks to others who have supported my pursuit of writing this book and my pursuit of competition:

My mom for being her beautiful self and telling me, "Sissy, jump out of *that airplane* while you can, before it's too late."

Bob Kinsey for his never-ending support of everything that I have pursued.

Avis Petty for always reminding me that God comes first.

John Turner and Paul Turner for technical support (and for being my friends).

Darla Sevieri for personal training and support throughout my competitions.

Terra Watson of DallasWear.net, Dallas, Texas, for designing all of my competition swimsuits and fitness costumes and pushing me to always be myself.

Jeff Johnson of FitnessMusic@aol.com for coordinating and compiling all of my fitness music and encouraging me to be Fifty, Fit, and Fabulous.

Girls Gone Wine and Creative Escapes (OK) for providing me with fantastic surroundings in which to pursue my writing career.

My new Toy Miniature Schnauzer, *Harley Spiderman Simmons*, for being by my side while I wrote my first book, ***Triple F: Fifty, Fit, and Fabulous.***

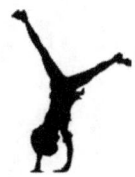

References

Agnew, Marion and Carly Burkhart. *Certified Personal Fitness Trainer & Nutritional Specialist (textbook)*. Ft. Collins: Weston Enterprises, 2005.

Bérubé, Sylvie, Caroline Diorio and Jacques Brisson. "Multivitamin-multimineral supplement use and mammographic breast density." *American Journal of Clinical Nutrition* (May 2008): 1400–404.

Blow, Steve. "At 91, woman goes after Addison City Council seat." *Dallas Morning News,* March 12, 2009.

Floyd, R. T. and Clem W. Thompson. *Manual of Structural Kinesiology, Fifteenth Edition*. New York: McGraw Hill Publishers, 2004.

Locke, E. A. and G. P. Latham. *A Theory of Goal Setting and Task Performance*. Upper Saddle River: Prentice-Hall, 1990.

www.whatittakes@runnersworld.com. "Finish 100 marathons at age 85." *Runners World Magazine*, March 2009: 22.

www.ingramcontent.com/pod-product-compliance
Lightning Source LLC
Chambersburg PA
CBHW060639290526
45793CB00001B/318